Praise for *India, My Calling*:

"Mary Haskett's latest book will enlighten and delight those who read it. Mary brings to life the story of Jean Darling, who as a young woman sets out on a two and a half month journey by land and sea, to serve as a missionary to India. Between a trying beginning and her return to Canada 40 years later, Jean's challenges and successes are vividly portrayed."

—Ruth Smith Meyer
Author of *Not Easily Broken*, *Not Far from the Tree*,
and *Tyson's Sad, Bad Day*

"The excellent story-telling skill of author Mary Haskett takes us on a charming and challenging journey with a real life heroine, missionary nurse, Jean Darling. Miss Darling's life of faith and courage will intrigue and entertain almost as much as it will inspire; Haskett's narrative and the 'letters home' written by Miss Darling transport us to another time and another place, where we see the goodness and the love of God manifested in and through the lives of his servants. *India My Calling* will be an inspiration to women of any age."

—Fay Rowe
Author of *What's in a Name*, *25,000 Mornings*,
and the award-winning *Keepers of the Testimony*

INDIA
MY CALLING

The Story of Jean Darling,

whose life work is in India

Mary Haskett

INDIA, MY CALLING
Copyright © 2012 by Mary Haskett

ISBN:978-1-77069-526-9

Printed in Canada.

Word Alive Press
131 Cordite Road, Winnipeg, MB R3W 1S1
www.wordalivepress.ca

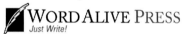

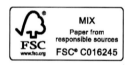

Library and Archives Canada Cataloguing in Publication

Haskett, Mary, 1934-
      India my calling / Mary Haskett.
ISBN 978-1-77069-526-9

          1. Haskett, Mary, 1934-. 2. Nurses--India--Biography.
3. Missionaries, Medical--India--Biography. 4. India--
Biography. 5. Nurses--Canada--Biography. I. Title.

R722.32.H38A3 2012   610.73092   C2012-901819-8

In this our fair land, there is much to do,
There is work for us all today
But to my own heart a call now has come
From a land that is far away.
There'll be many souls who'll perish in sin,
If you fail to show them the way.
My life and talents may seem to be
like the fishes and loaves so small.
But I have God's promise that He will bless.
So I give Him my best—my all.
Jean Darling, 1945

INDIA

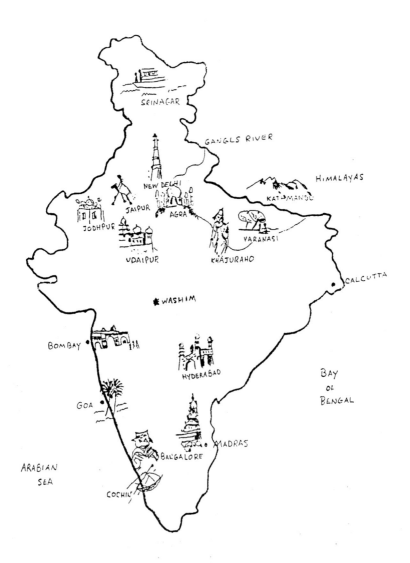

TABLE OF CONTENTS

तेव्हां
लोकसमुदायास
पाहून त्यांचा त्याला
कळवळा आला.

मात.९:३६
(MATH.९:३६)

ACKNOWLEDGEMENTS

For every author, I would surmise, there's a cheering team of family and friends.

My team took shape soon after I attended a birthday party almost two years ago. I met a lady there who told me she had enjoyed my book, *Reverend Mother's Daughter*. The lady then told me she knew of someone who also had a story worth telling. When she mentioned the name Jean Darling, I knew immediately who she was talking about. Jean Darling had been a missionary to India and from that faraway land had written letters to her family over a period of forty years. The family had kept all her letters and they had been tabulated by a friend, who hoped that someday, someone would write Jean's story.

"Would that friend be Pastor Rosalita Sorzano?" I asked. And yes, it was. Pastor Rose had shared with me months before about Jean and her letters.

So God set the wheels in motion, and soon I had in my possession the letters—stacks of them. Jean's descriptive style took me into another world. And like Pastor Rose, I saw a tale to be told.

Not every incident is related in this book, but enough to give the reader insight into the extraordinary life lived.

As I worked on Jean's story, a number of key players helped along the way. Jean herself, who I consulted with when I needed to verify facts. Audrey, Jean's wonderful sister, who is a continuous support to Jean and who has helped me in my quest to complete this project. And Pastor Rosalita Sorzano, whose enthusiasm has spurred me on.

I also thank my Ready Writer friends and fellow writers. And a special thanks to Ruth Smith Meyer and Fay Rowe for taking the time to read through the manuscript and make some suggestions.

And to Ray Wiseman, a member of the World Guild of Canada, who gave some early advice on where to begin. And to Shirley Howson for some early edits.

My church family, especially Janet and Theresa, and of course my pastors, Reverend Junior and Rosalita Sorzano.

And my children and grandchildren who have been interested in this project from the beginning and cheered when it was done.

To all of you, thank you.

And most of all, thanks be to God, who allowed its completion. As Jean says over and over again, "It's all to His glory."

INTRODUCTION

L ONG BEFORE MY HUSBAND, REVEREND JUNIOR SORZANO, AND I
became Jean Darling's pastors, we had heard stories about the
work of pioneer missionaries in India. While we were at Bible College
in Trinidad visiting missionaries, Reverend Bronell and Mrs. Greer
introduced us to Dr. Orpha Speicher's work and Reynolds Memorial
Hospital through the film *To Wipe a Tear*. However, when I came to
know Jean personally, missions in India came to life!

Jean's love of India and for "her people," as she called them, and her
passion for missions was obvious.

A few years after meeting Jean, she mentioned that on her return
from the mission field her family presented her with a large package.
They had kept all the letters she had written to them through the years.
I asked if I could read those letters, and quickly a seed was birthed in my
mind for a book.

A woman of unremarkable beginnings, Jean never felt that she was "specially gifted." To this day she is convinced that God can do amazing things through any person who will trust Him completely and serve Him wholeheartedly. However, I do believe that her life story is an example of what God can accomplish in and through ordinary people who are extraordinarily obedient. Her call was to start a nursing school in the Reynolds Memorial Hospital. Along with that she faced many dangers, cobras, rats and diseases. But her trust in God to take care of her through every circumstance never wavered.

Jean has always been interested in young people. She agreed to share her story with the hope that some young person will be challenged to answer God's call and discover the adventure of following and serving Jesus wherever He leads.

Recently, Jean gently corrected someone who noted that she must have brought many souls to salvation during her missionary career. Her gentle answer was, "I did not bring souls to Jesus. Jesus is the one who draws people to Himself. We are just instruments for His use."

As Jean nears the end of her earthly journey, she remains at peace—confident that "all is well." This remarkable woman continues to inspire us with her life of prayer and unshakable faith in her Saviour. She continues to bless us with her special gifts of encouragement, optimism and a life of heartfelt praise to God.

It is my privilege to know Jean Darling as friend, role model, mentor, and prayer warrior.

In Christ,
Reverend Rosalita Sorzano

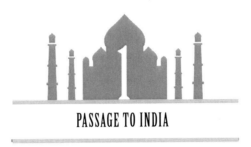

PASSAGE TO INDIA

THE RISE AND FALL OF THE WAVES STEADILY INCREASED AS THE STORM descended with ferocity in the coastal waters of Australia. The sea raged, sweeping mountainous white foam with relentless regularity over the decks of the Mulbera steamship. Jean Darling gripped the rails as she fought her way to the relative safety of her cabin. Salt spray stung her face. She could see Ruth ahead of her and shouted a word of encouragement, but the roaring wind carried her voice away.

A month previous, on October 16, 1945, the Matsonia, a passenger steamship, glided out of San Francisco Bay on its way to Australia. A slight evening breeze stirred. Jean, a twenty-six-year-old Canadian, stood on deck and watched lights that twinkled from the hilly terrain. She breathed a sigh of contentment as she considered the events that had brought her to this point.

It's like a dream, she thought. Four years ago, she had trained as a registered nurse in Victoria Hospital in London, Ontario, and now her desire, the inward urgency that had compelled her to apply to the Nazarene Headquarters for overseas service, was to be realized—God had called her to be a missionary to India.

The lights slowly disappeared and only the dark night remained. Jean and her travelling companion, evangelist Ruth Freeman, made their way to the seven-bunk cabin.

As they descended the steps, Jean reflected on her mother's influence in her life; her insistence in taking Jean, along with her brothers and sisters, to a series of evangelistic meetings in Grand Bend. The meetings, hosted by the Holiness Anderson Indiana movement, had left an indelible impression on Jean. Years later, as a young adult, she accepted an invitation to attend an evangelistic meeting in a United Church of Canada. Excitement flooded her heart at the thought of her salvation.

The women prepared for bed and Jean eyed the narrow upper bunk with a grin. "I hope I don't roll off," she said—but she did, landing with a loud thump. Groaning a little, she struggled up.

"What happened? Are you okay?" Ruth whispered.

"I think so." Jean straightened up and rubbed her shoulder, then put a hand to her head. "I'm still in one piece. Sorry about that."

She started to giggle, and that set Ruth off. But with a concentrated effort they settled down and Jean made sure she tucked her blanket in tight.

Although World War II had just ended and supplies were difficult to come by, food and service on the Matsonia were the very best. The nine-day voyage warranted a stop halfway. As the ship approached the island of Samoa in the Pacific Ocean, Jean stood on deck enthralled by the red and silver flying fish skidding along the surface of the sea, their colours radiant against the backdrop of a brilliant sunrise. Nearer to shore, she caught glimpses of palm trees, hills, and mountains displaying every shade of green imaginable. Soon the ship anchored in azure sea.

Samoa, a naval base, still housed many American servicemen. Deprived of visiting passenger ships for four years, they greeted the Matsonia with enthusiasm. With them were the islanders, whose ready smiles accentuated their dark skins. Their colourful wraparounds stood in stark contrast to the servicemen's uniforms.

Passengers disembarked for a few hours. Jean and Ruth, along with others, enjoyed a guided tour of the nearby village, where they watched women selling their crafts of woven mats, baskets, and colourful strung beads. Men also worked, preparing dough for bread which women cooked over wood fires. Jean wondered how India might compare to this tranquil scene.

The ship arrived in Brisbane on October 22. People crowded the dock waving flags and hats while a band played a rousing march. Mr. Sanner, a fellow traveler and Nazarene missionary, offered to assist the girls in retrieving their trunks. Noise and merriment dominated the jostling crowds.

"Stay close," Mr. Sanner yelled, as they made their way up the plank.

"Thank you so much." Jean clutched her hand luggage and did just that.

Once on the wharf, their benefactor secured the help of a deckhand to reclaim their trunks from the hold. Later they settled on a train that wended its way south to Sydney. The steady rhythm lulled Jean to sleep. After a while she awoke, thrilled to see kangaroos bouncing across the road.

On arrival in Sydney, the young women checked into the Glen Eagle Hotel where rooms had been booked for them. A strong smell of cigarette smoke and alcohol invaded their nostrils.

"Hello." A woman with very few teeth gave the girls a lopsided grin. "I'm the landlady," she announced with a liquid slur. "How can I help you?"

"Miss Freeman and Miss Darling," Ruth said. "We have a room booked here."

The landlady nodded. Her fingers moved with slow deliberation down a list of names on the desk.

"Follow me." She shuffled along the passageway and stopped at the bottom of the stairs, handing keys to Jean. "The first room on the left at the top. Bill will bring your luggage up. Dinner's at six."

MARY HASKETT

The girls entered a two-bedded room and glanced around to see faded quilts, curtains, and a small side table between the two beds. On it rested a rickety lampstand.

"Let's hope and pray we'll get a ship soon and be on our way to India," Jean said.

A knock on the door interrupted them. A large, red-faced man entered with their cases, plunked them down on the floor, and left.

Ruth lifted her case onto the bed and started to unpack. "You're right, Jean. We need to pray."

The next morning, a missionary couple who had also been booked into the hotel greeted Jean and Ruth in the dining room.

"How did you sleep?" Jean asked.

"We had a number of visitors," the woman said as she scratched at her arms.

"Us, too. I guess we've all been plagued by bedbugs."

"The customers in the bar didn't allow us much sleep. Take care when you go out. We heard some of them parting with their drink on the sidewalk."

Upstairs again, Jean and Ruth discussed their situation.

"We'll have to find other accommodation," Ruth said, "but it's going to be hard with all the people in town."

"You're right, but if we don't we'll make the best of it," Jean responded.

The young women made their way downtown, but soon learned rooms for rent were scarce. After the turmoil of World War II, Sydney had many evacuees, all trying to get back to their own countries. The girls decided to make the best of their situation, buying cereal, milk, and fruit for their breakfast. Many invites to homes and missionary gatherings eased their situation, and frequent trips down to the harbour looking for passage to India, or even a flight, kept them occupied.

On November 1, 1945, in the early morning, Jean sat at the small table in the bedroom. She took up her pen and began to write to her family. She told of their travels thus far, and went on to relate the difficulties they faced with the next step of the journey.

From Sydney

If we go by boat, it will be almost a month before we leave here. If by plane, maybe in a shorter time than that. I didn't realize that we would be having such a long stopover, but apparently Sarah Marquis, the agent in New York, did not let the National Missionary Council know about our coming, so the boat that is leaving on November 15 is full up. Anyway, it's freight and takes six weeks to get to India, since it stops at several places…we will probably have to go by cargo boat too, unless a passenger ship turns up…

The heat and the dubious sanitary conditions took their toll on Jean. Stomach cramps and vomiting were her lot at times. Undaunted, Jean determined to remain cheerful, and penned more news home, keeping a positive slant.

November 5, 1945, from Sydney

Two weeks have gone by since we came to Australia, and it has gone by so fast. I cannot imagine that I shall have been away from home five weeks…we are booked on a boat leaving November 13. We went to check again this morning and there was a cancellation. We are so glad about it, since God has answered our prayer. He can make ways where we cannot dream of it. However, we stop in Melbourne for nearly a week, from about the 15th to the 22nd, so we will not be really leaving Australia, although we shall sleep on the boat. It is a slow boat with stops in Perth, Ceylon, and then Calcutta and I don't know how many in-between.

I am enjoying the stay here, since now I am feeling fine again and it isn't as if I am alone, because God has been so precious and a wonderful friend these days.

The long-awaited voyage to India started in early November from Sydney. Jean wrote to her family, charting her progress aboard the steamship Mulbera as they sailed down the east coast to Melbourne.

Onboard the Mulbera

We left Sydney on November 16. We have Indians to make our beds, clean the floors, and bring us drinking water. They bring us tea and crackers at 6:15 am…They take our shoes and polish them. The food is very English-style, but we also have curry and rice like we will get in India. It is very good, and I know I will not starve. My face is getting fatter every day. I walk a lot on deck in the fresh air, and then sleep well all night. This trip is just what I needed. I have so much pep and feel I will be ready for work when I get to India. Although everything is strange, it is wonderful to know God and His peace in our hearts.

When they reached Melbourne, the ship docked for several days. Fifty missionaries disembarked, making their way to a reception held by the Mission Council. Here, the group shared with each other their areas of work on the mission field. Afterwards, they enjoyed some sightseeing.

With passengers back on board, the Mulbera made its way around the southern tip of Australia to Fremantle on the west coast. The ship docked a second time, and the passengers hurried into town to make some final purchases. Jean and Ruth bought bed nets and bicycle pumps—absolute necessities in India.

They sailed on. At first, Jean enjoyed the rise and dip of the waves. But a momentous storm was brewing. Passengers headed for their cabins. Jean stayed close behind Ruth as they staggered down the steps. Unable to stay upright, they bumped from side to side. They struggled on until they collapsed onto their narrow bunk beds, too exhausted to say a word. Jean felt the ship list so badly she began to wonder if they would be swallowed up into the foaming deep.

"Oh Lord," she prayed, "please keep us safe."

Their captain, with skill, fought to change course and move out of the storm's path, and after three days they sailed into calmer waters in the Indian Ocean on their way to Ceylon (Sri Lanka).

On day five, the ship anchored in Colombo Harbour. However, the vast number of boats left it some distance from the wharf. The passengers settled down to spend Christmas Day aboard the vessel. Jean and Ruth joined company with two other single women. They read their Bibles, prayed and exchanged small gifts. Jean prepared for bed around 1:30 am and, as she did, her stomach discomfort exacerbated into excruciating pain. Doubled over, she sat on the side of the bed and wrapped her arms around her middle.

"Oh, Ruth, what is it?" Jean gasped.

"I wish I knew. It could be a condition called 'chill in the tummy.' I read somewhere it can happen with climate change," Ruth said. "We're going to pray and then I'll get you a warm binder to wrap around your middle."

With relief, Jean felt the pain subside, and she slept.

She awoke the next morning desirous to keep going, looking forward with anticipation to the next step of the journey in spite of a residual nagging discomfort in her tummy.

The passengers were afforded a break before they journeyed on. So, along with other travelers, the girls were rowed ashore where they did more sightseeing and browsing stores. Back on board, Jean took up her pen and wrote:

December 26, 1945
The sunrises, the sunsets and the full moon make beautiful scenes, the most beautiful I've ever seen.

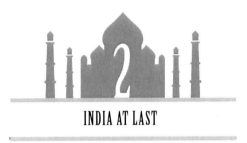

INDIA AT LAST

WITH RUTH AT HER SIDE, JEAN STRAINED TO SEE THE MANY SMALL craft on the water. She looked for any that might be headed toward their ship. They had arrived in Madras, the last port of call, and soon would step onto Indian soil.

She had received a letter in Colombo from Reverend Prescott Beals, Superintendent for the District. Reverend Beals, with twenty-five years on the mission field, had forged a strong fellowship for missionaries from the Nazarene churches and other denominations. He assured ongoing support, prayer meetings and retreats for them. He had written that he'd meet Jean and Ruth in Madras. Among the many boats on the water, she spotted a small rowboat with some white people in it. Having seen a picture of the Reverend Prescott Beals, she concentrated on the occupants to see if one of them might be him. Then much to her joy she heard a loud voice spell out BEALS.

With excitement, she and Ruth leaned over the rails, waving and shouting with vigour. "Here, here!"

A deckhand smiled at their enthusiasm. "We'll have him aboard in no time," he said.

The girls watched over the side as the gangway was lowered. Reverend Beals soon stepped aboard and warmly welcomed the new missionaries to India. They breakfasted together and, after police and custom formalities, they, with help from crew members, carefully traversed the gangway and settled into the rowboat that headed for land.

The cacophony of sound and the swirling tide of human beings and the clamouring of brown hands begging for money created chaos on the wharf. Children and adults alike begged. "Candy, candy," the children cried, as they held up their hands in anticipation. One little girl, her hair hanging about her face, wore worn-out sandals a size too big; she was more bent on earning money. She insisted Jean's shoes needed polishing and finally she won out—her reward two cents. With a smile on her face, she pushed the money into a small cloth bag hanging around her neck.

The porters who carried their bags haggled over how much the missionaries should pay them. Jean observed Brother Beals, quiet and firm, handle the situation with aplomb. He secured a taxi and they were taken to Central Station, where they deposited their heavy luggage.

Brother Beals had booked rooms in the American Baptist Rest Home, and there they stayed for a few days, only going out to buy more necessities for their final destination. This included bedrolls and pillows, which they were to take with them wherever they went; also topees—lightweight sun helmets.

"All your drinking water has to be boiled," Brother Beals said, as he directed them into a store to purchase metal water canteens. These, they learned, were to be slung on their backs like knapsacks.

Back at the rest house, their purchases completed, the superintendent advised the women to go to bed early, since they had a long train journey the next day.

"I am ready for bed," Jean announced, as they made their way to the bedroom.

"Me too," Ruth said, confirming the admission with a loud yawn.

Ablutions completed, within minutes they were fast asleep.

Jean suddenly awoke, startled by a loud clanging and the sound of many voices. She sat bolt upright.

"Ruth, do you hear that?"

"Yes. What is it?"

The girls stumbled out of bed and crept over to the window. Pulling back the curtains, they saw a vast number of Indian people. Children, men, and women in bright saris waved banners. They marched down the middle of the street singing, and great joy exuded from their faces.

"They're Christians," Jean whispered, as she recognized a familiar hymn. "How exciting. It must be their New Year's Eve service." They watched and listened for a while, then decided to go back to bed. Sleep eluded them for most of the night, as the crowd sang on into the wee hours.

A pair of weary young ladies made their way down to breakfast the next morning. Brother Beals explained there had been four languages used in the festivities: Hindustani, Telegu, Tamil and English. He smiled. "Well, a happy new year to you both, and may God bless you as you labour for Him in India. We have to leave for the train station directly after breakfast. I'll arrange for a taxi and meet you at the front door."

But on New Year's Day 1946, no taxis were available. "We will have to go by rickshaw," Brother Beals said. He stepped onto the sidewalk and flagged down three. Jean grinned at the novelty as the young men with a steady trot pulled them to Central Station.

They entered the vast and impressive building, evidence of British architecture, and made their way to the ticket counter.

"No sir, no more accommodation," the ticket master announced, as he waved both hands in the air. "You take first class if you like. First class is very good sir."

"We have no choice," Brother Beals said to the girls, and he bought tickets. Arrangements were made to have their luggage taken from storage and placed on the train.

They followed the porter along the platform and saw that people stood shoulder to shoulder in the compartments. The first-class accommodation presented a very different scenario. The young women were ushered into a compartment with plush seats and bunk beds.

"This is amazing," Jean remarked, as she peered into a bathroom complete with shower.

"Evidence of the British influence," Brother Beals said, as they settled in their seats.

The train pulled slowly out of the station, gradually gathering speed. Jean viewed the landscape with a keen eye. She noted rice fields, small mud huts slung low to the ground with straw roofs, people washing clothes in rivers and muddy pools, and numerous temples, some stately and impressive, others in disarray.

Over a timeframe of thirty-one hours, the train stopped several times en route to Akola, and on each occasion people crowded at the windows begging for money. "Buckshee, buckshee," they cried, pressing their hands together as if praying, then opening them to receive whatever might be given.

The group transferred to Reverend Beals' Studebaker for the seventy-mile drive to Chikhli, where the missionary resided with his wife. They shared the dirt road with Indians travelling on foot, on bicycles, in carts, and pulling carts. As evening approached, wagons pulled by oxen appeared on the road, loaded with cotton.

"They bring the cotton in at evening time," Brother Beals said, as he mopped his brow with a handkerchief. "It allows some relief for the poor beasts from the intense heat of the day."

"Is that small girl really picking up cow manure?" Jean asked.

Brother Beals laughed and then explained. Later, Jean wrote in one of her letters,

> …They dry it and use it for fuel, for not one part of the sacred cow can be wasted. Also they wet it and plaster it all over the floor, smooth it and pat it down with their hands…

On January 2, 1946, the party arrived at the Beals' home. Mrs. Beals greeted them warmly. "Come in, my dears. Rahul will take the luggage to your rooms."

Mrs. Blackman, a fellow missionary from Basim, which would be home base for the women, handed Jean twenty-three letters. "Your family has written regularly during your voyages."

Ruth and Jean were in for a blessing when they learned the Beals had delayed Christmas dinner until their arrival. All the missionaries from the district attended.

In her next letter home, Jean wrote:

> …We had a good time and felt so much at home here. The bungalow is large and spacious and is furnished very nicely. Of course, the Beals have been here for twenty-five years…We had peacock fowl for Christmas dinner. It was delicious. …Brother Beals told me to give all of you his best wishes for the new year…he is a wonderful man. In fact, all of our missionaries are lovely. Doctor Speicher had to go away on business, so I haven't met her yet, but will tomorrow…

The next day, she and Ruth journeyed on to their final destination—the Reynolds Memorial Hospital in Basim. Jean knew about Doctor Orpha Speicher, a remarkable woman of God who served as the sole physician at the hospital, which had at one time been a school. The Nazarenes had purchased it in 1934 in derelict condition. Doctor Speicher had the foresight to see its potential. With persistent fundraising and determination, she envisioned the building, outhouses, and bungalows as a vibrant medical complex. Basic work had been started, with garbage swept away, the mud floors scrubbed, and the walls whitewashed. However, the ultimate goal was yet to be achieved.

Although other missionary nurses had preceded Jean, she knew her own mission had a special mandate. In order to fulfill it, she needed to become familiar with the Indian way of life and learn the language of the region—Marathi. Bubbling with excitement at every new encounter she experienced, she looked forward to more.

Their car journey ended. Brother Beals pulled into the sprawling complex of the Reynolds Memorial Hospital, and stopped in front of one of three bungalows.

"Hello, Kissen," he called out to a man, who came across the courtyard.

"Welcome, welcome," the man said. With hands pressed together, he bowed and smiled.

Everyone trooped into the bungalow. Brother Beals had told the girls that they would share the accommodation with Doctor Speicher. Jean looked around. She listened as Kissen, in broken English, related the story of a servant killing a cobra just across the road from the bungalow the day before. She watched as Brother Beals placed his arm around Kissen's shoulders and spoke in the Marathi language. The simple gesture of brotherly love moved her. The two laughed together and then proceeded to unload the luggage.

God, thank you for bringing me here. May I learn the language quickly and be a blessing in this place, Jean silently prayed.

There were many new situations to face, not least among them a conglomerate of animal species, including huge black ants, scorpions, and monkeys everywhere, all part of what to see and expect in her new environment.

With enthusiasm, she wrote of her first experiences:

…It is wonderful to have such a big bedroom with bed, dressers, wardrobe, bookcase, a lovely big desk, a little table and three chairs. The ceilings are very high and the windows are high too, so the rooms are very bright and we don't need curtains.

From now on there will be welcome services for us at each station in the district, then we get down to language study with a private teacher for a while, and then we go to language school about February 15 at Mahableshwar for three months. It is a hill station and it's cool up there…

Dressed in saris, the traditional Indian dress, the girls experienced their first welcome service. Graduates from the Bible College preached in Marathi, and Jean gave it her full attention, listening to the cadence of the language as well as the interpreter. The service ended with Indian girls placing a garland of flowers around their necks and presenting them with a bouquet. Jean marveled at the exquisite beauty of the Indian girls, and later wrote of it in a letter to her family.

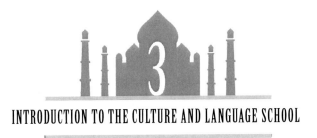

INTRODUCTION TO THE CULTURE AND LANGUAGE SCHOOL

WITH A CHEERFUL SMILE, DOCTOR SPEICHER APPROACHED JEAN, who sat at a small table in the outpatient clinic. "We're going on a mission," she said.

Jean closed her notebook. She had been working on a nursing curriculum. Together, the two left the complex of the Reynolds Memorial Hospital.

There's still much work to be done, Jean thought as they passed the whitewashed walls. Still, on this January day in 1946, she followed the lone doctor into the courtyard.

Jean resolved to increase the nursing staff from one to many. She planned to train girls from the villages in nursing skills and techniques. She felt a surge of excitement at the thought as she and Doctor Speicher, with the help of the driver, climbed into the cumbersome cart pulled by oxen.

The animals ambled along over rough terrain, causing bumps and jolts. They arrived on the outskirts of a small village situated some fifteen miles from the hospital. As they clambered down from the cart, they were greeted with shouts of "Salaam," meaning peace.

"Stay close to me, Jean," Doctor Speicher said.

Entering a gateway, they trudged along narrow alleys. Villagers followed them, their high-pitched chatter dominating the air. From a school, Jean heard the shouts of children. *This is how they study, all talking or singing at once,* she later wrote in one of her letters. Soon, they came to a village surrounded by tall mud walls. The oppressive heat caused Jean to wipe her face more than once.

"We're here to help a mother in labour," Doctor Speicher said.

A man came out of one of the homes and chatted excitedly to Doctor Speicher, beckoning her to follow. "It seems the mother has already delivered," she told Jean. "We'll check her anyway."

Jean peered over the doctor's shoulder and could make out dozens of people in the dark interior. Doctor Speicher, speaking loudly, told them to wait outside. The tone of her voice caused them to understand, since they were Hindus and she wasn't completely versed in their language yet. With much chit-chat, they exited. Jean could not see a thing, except for the tiny glow of a candle in the corner. The room was so stuffy she could hardly breathe. She strained to see the husband and eventually saw that he was kneeling beside a mattress on the floor. His wife lay there moaning softly as she cradled a tiny baby in her arms.

Doctor Speicher pulled out a flashlight and examined the mother while she spoke to her gently. She administered treatment and then examined the baby. This done, she indicated to the husband that she wanted to talk to him, and he followed into the bright sunlight.

Writing to her family of the incident, Jean wrote:

> …We came out and sat on a bench, while Doctor Speicher explained to the family when to give medication and how. But finally they had to call the school master because no one could understand. Then they brought hot milk with oodles of sugar and spices for us to drink. It is an insult and dishonour

not to drink it, so we did. About fifty people stood, sat and listened to everything Doctor Speicher had to tell them. It was an opportunity to tell them about Christ, who saves from sin. There had never been a preacher or worker in that village before.

This morning I went out to a village with four Indian Christian ladies. We left at 8:30 am and sat down in front of several houses. The ladies sang and talked, and about thirty people came around and sat down to listen. The monkeys were jumping around from trees to the houses and then back and forth. I thought one might land on my topee (sun hat) but it did not. The ladies also took me into the stores where they sold saris. They taught me some new words, and it was surprising how one can use a few words and expressions she knows. I had a great time!

"Mind the steps, they are very steep. Our legs are going to be aching by the time we get to the top," Doctor Speicher said.

Following close behind, Jean wondered if the steps before them could be any worse than the dark alley they had just navigated.

"They're a great family," Doctor Speicher said. "I'm praying for their salvation."

It soon became clear they couldn't climb the steps and converse, and only their laboured breathing could be heard as they ascended.

A voice called out from the top of the stairs. "Velcome, velcome, Doctor Speicher."

They entered a big bright room. Their hostess greeted them graciously and welcomed Jean into her home. Two little girls peeped from behind their mother's skirts, watching Jean with some curiosity. Their mother spoke to them and they ran from the room giggling.

"Please sit," she said, indicating a mattress on the floor. "I will bring sweets for you." And so she did on a brass tray.

As Jean looked up to take some food, movement on the beam above caught her eye. She gulped—two or three rats were scuttling back and forth. Their hostess said, "Please eat. They will not bother us."

Concentrating on the tray, Jean told herself that the rats appeared to be busy with their own activities so why should she be concerned? She prayed silently, smiled at the hostess, took a plate, and helped herself to a sweet dessert. She didn't care for it very much, so decided it was better to eat it quickly. The hostess mistook her motive and insisted she have more, piling her plate high. *Oh my, a lesson learned*, she thought.

On their way back, Jean told Doctor Speicher about her ongoing health issues.

"I'm afraid you have amoebic dysentery," Doctor Speicher said. "You will have to take antibiotics and saline treatments."

As well as the physical problem, more than half of Jean's belongings that she had shipped to India had been stolen en route to Basim. In spite of her trials, she said to Doctor Speicher, "Material things come and go, but there is one thing He gives that no one can take away."

Lying on her bed, too weak to engage in any activity, Jean prayed, "Oh Lord, you know I'd rather be with Ruth and Paula in language school. Please help." She had suffered a bout of the debilitating disease for ten days and had no recourse but to lie low. On the eleventh day of this particular episode, she decided she had to get to language school whatever her condition, and in the middle of March she got up, packed, and, with the help of a servant, started the three-and-a-half day journey to Mahableshwar, a village situated high in the mountains a hundred miles south of Bombay. Here she joined Ruth and Paula, a specialist in education. They were housed in a bungalow called The Cliff.

The young women started the day with a fifteen-minute walk to school for one hour of class. Returning to the house, they had another hour of instruction on a one-to-one basis.

Soon after Jean's arrival, Ruth, Paula and Jean compared notes in their bungalow. Jean remarked, "Two hours is quite enough for me. I'll be so glad when I'm free of this pesky bug. It makes me so tired." She sighed and looked at her roommates with a rueful smile. "I'd like to eat a hearty meal without having to think about what I'm eating. I just love curry and rice. Too bad it has to be off my diet."

Ruth gave her arm a squeeze. "I'm sure you'll soon be healed, Jean."

Later, Jean sat at the small table in their bedroom, stared out of the window for a moment, viewing the beauty of the mountains, and then took up her pen and wrote:

> …Since I left home, many have been the experiences and many the sights. Many have been the disappointments and many the joys, but I'm glad that with each step Jesus leads and makes a way…with all this comes the experience of drawing closer to the One who meets all our needs, who blesses our souls to overflowing and keeps us in His care, while He fills our hearts with joy unspeakable, and full of Glory…

"Hi, Jean. Can I talk to you?" Ruth stood in the doorway.

"Sure. I've just finished my letter."

"Since you will be housekeeper next week, I want to go over a few things with you. As you know, many Indians are ignorant of even basic hygiene, and side streets and fields are used to dispense with bodily waste, which means we have to make sure the Indian servants allotted to us wash their hands thoroughly. We've been showing them how to soak the vegetables and fruit in salt water and boil all the water." Ruth frowned. "I can tell you, it's a challenge. One thing we discovered is that the vendors in the bazaar water down the milk and sometimes add powdered potato to make it look creamy."

"So you're telling me to be on the alert when we go to buy produce."

"That's right. But meanwhile we pray and trust God to help us be good witnesses."

Jean settled into her stint as housekeeper and pressed on with her language studies. Her physical discomforts persisted, but still she remained true to the task before her. Finally, on March 30, 1946, almost six months after leaving Canada, Jean received word her tests had come back negative for amoebic dysentery. The colitis caused by the disease created episodes of pain, and she had to continue a diet of strained foods for a while.

The dry season, starting in April, generated untold suffering for the population. Rumours of a pending famine began to dominate the news of the day, and it was estimated millions of Indians could be affected. *The Times of London,* on March 25, 1946, reported:-

> The drought in India has caused a food shortage of dimensions which as the government has realized, necessitate a full mobilization of resources in men, and money, and machines, in administrative energy and resourcefulness, and in political influence to save millions of Indians from starvation.

Along with this pending catastrophe, political unrest loomed. Stirred by Mahatma Gandhi, millions of Indians joined him in rallies seeking independence from Britain. This became the catalyst for Britain ceding and the proposed partitioning of India, with Pakistan coming into its own. The suggested divide created much unrest between Mohammadens (Muslims), Hindus, minority groups, the state of Hyderabad, and its rulers and nobles. Hyderabad wished to align with Pakistan, which created a huge problem, since the New Union of India surrounded it completely. This state of affairs brought about the rumblings of civil war and fighting between the differing groups.

It was to this environment that Jean and her companions had come. They wondered if their mission work could proceed, or if they might be instructed to return home. As the girls walked in the hills in reflective thought, Jean spoke.

"I hope after learning this language we will be able to go back down to the plains and start our mission work. I loved those few weeks in Basim before we came up here to Mahableshwar, and I love the people. I'm so looking forward to seeing them all again."

"Me too," Ruth said.

They returned to the bungalow to find more parcels of canned foods, chocolate and home-baked cakes had arrived.

"It amazes me the way these parcels get through," Jean said. She stood at the window and looked at distant mountains shrouded in mist, and closer ones green and lush. *Such beauty*, she thought, *and all around us turmoil.* In the far distance she could hear another political rally taking place in the centre of the village, and at the same time the wailing sound of bagpipes floated up to the bungalow. "Another wedding," she remarked. "Four days of bagpipes again, mingled with the Congress Party rallies. Oh well, this is India."

"You're right," Ruth intoned. "Not only that, if you ever get married you better not do it Indian-style. I don't want bagpipes playing for four days." The girls laughed.

In the evening, their studies finished, Jean tidied up the sitting room and Ruth made her way to the bedroom. The quiet suddenly shattered as Jean heard Ruth let out a piercing scream.

"What is it?" Jean went to her friend's bedside to see a lizard caught in the netting. "That's all?" She grinned. "Another critter for my collection." With that she scooped up her butterfly net and deftly caught the little creature, depositing it in a tin box on the desk.

Their time in language school and their rigorous study drew to a close. On May 22, 1946, the girls had a four-day break and decided to read from Ruth's Marathi Bible the gospel of Mark, before taking a walk down to the bazaar. On the Thursday, Jean wrote again to her family:

…This has been an interesting week thus far. Monday and Tuesday we had a holiday from our private hour, so had much less homework. Tuesday morning Ruth and I went to the bazaar, and just as we got onto the main street, there was a parade of about fifteen men, and one of them threw money all over the street. We looked and looked. It was a funeral parade! There were four men carrying a canvas stretcher bound with straw and the corpse was bound on that. It was all covered with bright orange cloth. We followed them. Our coolie said it would be okay. Two boys were beating drums and they walked very fast while wailing and crying, "Rama, Rama, suthe she," which means Rama, Rama, he is the true god. On the way to the place of burning, they put the body on the ground, put some kind of sugar in her hand (for it was a woman) and marched around bowing and worshipping. Then when we got to the place, they took off her jewels and swept a spot on the ground, put fresh cow dung on it to purify it and then sprinkled water on that to complete the process. Then they piled up wood in the shape of a coffin and rolled her onto it face down and covered her up with more wood, until she could not be seen…they put dry cow dung and coconuts among the wood. The only mourner was her son, for women in India are too afraid to go to a funeral. He ran around the pile with a lighted straw to start the fire and then another man took over. It surely was a sight to see, but it was terrible to realize that one more of India's millions went to eternity without God…I want more than ever to lead souls to Christ. We thought we would never see such a sight again, but this morning while going to school we met another procession. It was different from the other and conducted by a priest. The body was not covered, she wore a dress for it was a woman too, and her mouth was wide open. The Hindus burn their dead, the Mohammedans bury theirs, and the Parsi, a minority group, with roots in Iran, put theirs on big rafters and the vultures eat the corpses, then the bones are put through some purifying process…

"What a vast and diverse culture I'm in," Jean murmured as she finished typing. She sealed the letter and called out to Paula and Ruth, "How about a Victoria buggy ride and some sightseeing before we go to Satara District?"

Ruth came into the living room and sat down on the couch. "I'm all for it," she said.

Their afternoon excursion took them to old Mahableshwar, where they visited a number of temples. Some of the temples had a large bull at the entrance and indicated that they worshiped the cow. Many statues of goddesses and gods were situated at the temple sites where persons were designated to wash them at certain times and to tend the flower gardens surrounding them.

Jean spoke in a low voice. "My, how can people be so misinformed? We have a huge task before us. God help us to share His love."

Back at the bungalow, Jean announced, "Time for our shots." With that, they administered cholera and typhoid injections to each other—

an absolute necessity with the hoped-for rainy season approaching. Language school now over, they spent the rest of the evening packing, for they were to leave for the Satara District the next day.

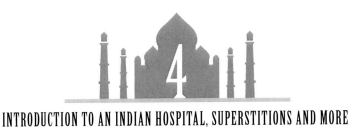

INTRODUCTION TO AN INDIAN HOSPITAL, SUPERSTITIONS AND MORE

I n the Wai Christian Hospital halfway up the Himalayas in the Sarata District, Jean stood and listened to a doctor in conversation with a patient who had a growth on her leg. The doctor shook his head and turned to Jean.

"She has had it for ten years and has been putting guinea feathers around it, believing her gods would heal it," he said. He spoke kindly to the woman and explained he would operate on her leg and remove the growth. Gripped with fear and superstition, her husband insisted on staying in the operating room. The doctor explained to him that his wife would be fine and he could stay with her as soon as she came out of surgery.

He turned to Jean. "You will see whole families coming in and setting up like campers under the beds of the patients. So be prepared," he added with a smile.

The surgery completed, Jean went to the outpatient area, where she observed a seasoned missionary nurse dealing with the patients coming into the clinic—among them several mothers with desperately sick babies.

"Why are the babies so thin and lethargic?"

The nurse looked at Jean. "You have much to learn. The babies are a huge concern for us, and we pray the mothers will trust God. They fear coming here and hang onto their superstitions until their babies are almost at death's door. The mothers work in the fields all day. Unfortunately, because they have no one to care for their babies, they feed them opium before they leave."

"Opium!" Jean exclaimed.

"Yes, the baby stays in a semi-comatose state all day. We have a baby over there whose leg has been chewed away, most likely by a rat."

These somber scenarios once again brought home to Jean the great need for the gospel in India. She longed to get back to Basim—to home, as she liked to call the place where she would live and work.

Introduction into hospital procedure completed, Jean travelled to Bombay with Ruth and Paula. Although the rainy season had started, intense heat and humidity persisted. Brother Beals and his wife met them upon arrival, looking a little more comfortable in the heat than the girls.

"We're going to take you on a sightseeing excursion," Mrs. Beals said. This included a visit to a Parsi burial ground, that minority group that laid its dead on high constructions to be devoured by vultures. The visit over, they enjoyed the beauty and diversity of Bombay, browsing stores with a vast array of wares. Among other items, Jean purchased a Marathi Bible and some canned foods, then the young women returned to Basim.

"One thing I realize," Jean remarked, as the train rattled along. "We only have a basic knowledge of Marathi and much more study has to be done before we master the language."

Her companions nodded in agreement.

Settled again in Basim, Jean wrote to her parents:

> …It is wonderful to sleep on my new bed and to be back home again. All the people in the village look so good. I never

realized one could miss them so much. I have been looking forward to coming back to the plains…

She sealed her letter and hurried across the Reynolds Memorial Hospital grounds to the outpatient clinic. More packages had arrived from church support groups, and she knew they contained much-needed items of sheets, pillow cases, bandages and clothing for babies and adults. She hoped to get the items unpacked before patients started to arrive. She stepped into the clinic and Doctor Speicher greeted her.

"We have a very sick baby, Jean. We'll have to take care of it now. Can you bring a sterile tray and gowns?"

Jean nodded. She hurried to the clinic room and gathered the equipment. She passed patients waiting to be seen, and called out that she'd be with them soon.

The baby did not have veins viable enough to insert a needle. "We'll try hypo- alimentation," Doctor Speicher said. She gently inserted a hypodermic needle just under the skin into the wasted muscle. Jean attached the tubing, hung the IV bottle on the stand and opened the drip.

"Let's try this for twelve hours," Doctor Speicher suggested, "then we can see if he's strong enough to take fluid from an eyedropper. The very best we can do is pray," she added. "Diphtheria is not good in such a tiny infant."

The women dispensed with their gowns and masks. Doctor Speicher spoke with kindness to the mother and explained the gravity of the illness.

The baby did not survive, and his tearful mother wrapped the body and took it away.

Jean worked with Doctor Speicher nonstop for weeks. Patients clamoured into the outpatient area with fevers, sores, and wounds to be tended, patients with sinuses—holes in their muscles where flesh-eating worms had burrowed, and patients with gangrenous limbs, due to ignorance.

Then news came that a breakout of bubonic plague had surfaced in the village. Doctor Speicher reported the matter to the district health officer. As the news spread, the villagers packed up their belongings and headed out to the fields where they set up camp in order to get away from the flea-infested rats that carried the disease. The Bible students, dressed in special clothing and makeshift masks, volunteered to go into the village and spray each home with DDT powder. They worked for days and became a witness of God's love.

Doctor Speicher ordered anti-plague vaccine from Bombay. Everyone who came to the hospital—police, business persons, patients—was stopped outside the compound, sprayed with DDT and given the injection and a certificate confirming the treatment. Jean, Doctor Speicher, and other missionaries went out in teams of two and administered 19,000 injections to the villagers camped in the fields. Twenty-two villages had been infected. The scripture that came to Jean during those tumultuous days resonated in her mind as she went about the work: *"There shall no evil befall thee, neither shall any plague come nigh thy dwelling"* (Psalm 91:10).

Back in the hospital, Jean talked to a young mother as she huddled her sick child to her breast. "You bring all your family for injection. It will be good for you and keep the sickness away." The advice slowly registered with the villagers, and many came to the clinic for prophylactic treatments.

The nursing school often popped into Jean's mind, and she prayed that God would soon send students. The churches and Christian community had spread the word that a nurse had come to teach. One day, as she bandaged a patient's arm, she noticed a group of girls come into the clinic. They stood talking quietly among themselves. Her task finished, she went to speak to them.

"We would like to be nurses," a girl with a beautiful smile said. "We heard at church that you will teach us."

Overjoyed, Jean set a date with the girls.

At supper that night, she announced to Doctor Speicher, "My nursing school starts next Monday."

"Wonderful," the doctor beamed. "What a difference it will make to have a body of trained nurses." Jean prayed that over the weekend, the clinic would remain quiet so she could go over her already prepared curriculum of practical and pediatric nursing, obstetrics and medical, plus outpatient services. She smiled as she thought about the method of teaching, knowing her limited knowledge of the language could be a stumbling block. Unruffled, she determined visual aid would be paramount.

Under a tree in the courtyard, where early morning chapel took place, the first group of student nurses commenced classes on a June morning. During the rainy season, classes were to be held in the outpatient department. Jean secured the services of a tailor to make uniforms for the girls. This approach instilled pride and purpose into the class and caused diligent study. Meanwhile, spurred on by the response, Jean concentrated on her own study of the language and incorporated its use into her lectures.

"Don't forget to always use forceps when doing sterile dressings." Jean watched as one of her students demonstrated the sterile technique on a patient with an ulcerated leg and correctly applied the dressing. "Good, good." She smiled, showing her approval. "I appreciate we've had to use very basic techniques to prepare these instruments. Boiling an enamel kettle in the courtyard and placing our instruments in it is not the ideal. But it will do until we get sterilizers installed. Well, girls, back to your duties, and do review the handouts on sterile techniques."

Sterile techniques were uppermost in her mind. The use of cow manure by the Indians for every conceivable ailment was a huge challenge to overcome. Women in the villages smeared cow dung all over the pregnant mothers in order to hasten delivery. They came into the hospital with festering, putrid wombs, all because of ignorance and false gods. Many of the mothers died and a building in the hospital grounds became home to the babies who survived. They were cared for by an Indian Christian lady. The nursing students were agents of change for healthy lifestyles; they were part of the ministry team to spread the good news of the gospel to those who came under their care.

"Greetings, Sister."

Jean looked up to see Ambibai Manmothe coming towards her. She stopped and watched Ambibai, who walked slowly with a cane.

"How are you today?" Jean asked

"Well, well," the old lady said, her eyes bright and full of love. They entered the hospital together. "I wonder how many today."

Jean marveled at the faithfulness of the little lady, who came to the hospital each day to tell patients and their relatives about Jesus. Everyone knew her as the Bible woman. Jean recalled how she had first met Ambibai. She had been resting along the side of the road when Jean happened by. Ambibai told Jean how Jesus had come to her in a vision and shown her a field full of wheat. She had said to Jesus, "I am very tired. I have brought to you many sheaves. Could I quit now?"

Jesus replied, "Yes, my child, you have brought many sheaves, but there are so many still to be gathered in. You cannot quit now." And so Ambibai carried on. Eventually they found a bed for her, and she lived out her days on the ward.

On August 15, Jean again pulled out her typewriter; only the clicking of the keys could be heard as she wrote to her family once more:

> ...I feel fine except I am very tired as usual. All the missionaries are exhausted by the time night comes, so don't think that it is unusual for me to be so tired. We can hardly make it to 1:30 pm or 2:00 pm when we can go to bed for a rest in the afternoon. Doctor S has been sick; we both ate something that upset us last Saturday night. I was never so sick to my stomach in my life.
>
> On Sunday we had two babies born and one operation. I delivered one of the babies and she other...Today Doctor S did not go to clinic, so I saw all the patients, wrote down the symptoms, then came up to the bungalow with their cards. She wrote down the treatments. It is very hard to understand what they are saying, and it is very tiring having to concentrate all the time and listen so carefully...I am like a rag afterward. Here they speak Marathi and Hindi. I'm glad I have a little bit of music in me—it helps me to detect the various sounds. I'm glad I took music, for now I realize it was God's leading...it is invaluable.

Jean finished her letter by commenting on the most recent news she had received from her family. She checked her watch and decided to go over to the hospital. As Jean entered the outpatient department, a woman wearing a rich colourful silk sari spoke to her.

"My child is very sick. Can you help?"

Jean recognized her as a woman of wealth from the village. She examined the child and gave her medication, since Doctor Speicher had gone out on a house visit. Although she felt some qualms about the whole matter, she prayed her prescription would work. The grateful mother came back three days later with a well child and much praise for Jean.

Doctor Speicher needed to attend the district and other meetings at times, and with a capable nurse holding the fort she was able to do so. On a quiet afternoon, Jean checked the inpatients, and noted all were comfortable. As she walked across the courtyard, she turned at the sound of loud, agitated voices coming from the outpatient department. She hurried back to see a woman carried by a man, her head lolled back, and she pale, her sari bloodied.

"What happened?"

"A wild boar, Sister. A wild boar attacked her."

"Come." Jean had the woman placed on a cot. On examination, she observed a number of open wounds on her arms and legs and in her side. They had travelled a long distance and the heat had not helped. The stench of rotting flesh was almost unbearable. With the assistance of a student nurse, she cleaned and packed the wounds. Again she realized the patient needed to start antibiotic treatment immediately. Without hesitation she prepared an injection of penicillin. She silently thanked God for the Methodist Mission who supplied them with medications. For three days and nights she hardly slept, dressing and packing the wounds and giving penicillin injections every six hours.

When Doctor Speicher returned, her patient's overall condition had improved, but the arm could not be saved, and Doctor Speicher had to amputate. In spite of this, the patient made a good recovery. In her next letter home, Jean wrote, "*The Lord is good to help me when these cases come in.*"

By December of that year, Jean wrote her language exams. With excitement, she wrote to her family:

> I passed my exams with honours, but do not know the exact mark. There were seventeen who tried the exam and two of us got honours. One failed all exams and three failed part of the exam. Ruth passed, too. I thought I had done poorly because I was so scared, but the convener of the language school sent me my certificate and told me that my oral exam was especially good and they could not believe I had only been studying for ten months. Please don't tell anyone this, or they will think I'm just tooting my own horn. I was very pleased, but realize many people were praying for me and the Lord helped me a great deal.

Jean stopped writing for a moment, as her thoughts turned to Brother Beals. He had been visiting the hospital for a few days, as his responsibilities dictated. Now he lay in one of the bungalows, having contracted diphtheria. Although he was on the mend, he would return home to Chikhli and be on bed rest for two more weeks, which meant Christmas Day in bed. She thought of Agnes, a missionary in the district, slated for surgery, and of her own health struggles with stomach upsets. She prayed for them all, then closed her letter.

Toward the end of the week, Jean sat in the courtyard and wrote her last letter of the year:

> December 27, 1946
> Dear Mom and all,
> We had a lovely Christmas here. I expect you had a good time, too. In India, one really realizes the true meaning of Christmas. The Indian people have a lot of celebration for about a week…last Monday afternoon, the children and mothers celebrated. They came to the Bible School and received gifts of cloth from the mission. For all the Christian children cloth is rationed and they can hardly get enough to wear. On Monday,

a concert was put on by the day school children (an ordinary school). There were three hundred people and mostly non-Christians. It was an opportunity to tell them of the birth of our Lord Jesus Christ...

Jean described the events that had taken place on Christmas Eve, of tea served to the elderly ladies in the village, of the church people putting on a play about the birth of Jesus, and how many Hindus and Mohammedans attended. She shared how the missionaries secured a tree, trimmed it to the shape of a Christmas tree and added a sprinkling of soap flakes to make it look like snow! She told more:

...We went to bed about twelve midnight, and at 12:30 am, the nurses came singing Christmas carols. That is the custom here to sing all night and go from place to place. They came around to everyone's window and sang. Doctor Speicher got up and gave them candy. I got up and wished them merry Christmas and thanked them for coming. I was thrilled. Then, at 3:30 am, the Bible School boys parked at our front veranda and sang and beat the drums, until I finally got up and gave them candy and then they went away...

As she finished her letter, Jean gazed across the courtyard and wondered what 1947 might bring.

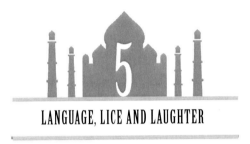

LANGUAGE, LICE AND LAUGHTER

CARE OF THE SICK NEVER CEASED AND JEAN LOVED IT, EVEN THOUGH exhaustion plagued her at times. Under Doctor Speicher's leadership, renovations and additions continued to improve the standard in the hospital and surrounding buildings. Rooms and a kitchen were added to the bungalow. The American army had donated three of their vehicles to the work of the mission, including an ambulance. More and more, Jean saw God's hand upon their endeavors. In her January letter, she wrote:

> ...I often think about you all and wish I could just drop in and then come back. I would never change the experiences of this past year for anything in the world. I really love the work and will like it even more when I can work full-time and not have to worry about passing exams...

At the beginning of March, Jean set out for Mahableshwar with Ruth, Paula, and other missionaries and servants—the journey long, hot and tiring. When they reached Poona, there were no hotel rooms available, so they spent the night sleeping on benches in the railway station—at least on the benches, but no sleep, since they were attacked by bedbugs. Jean welcomed the morning gratefully as they boarded a train to Mahableshwar, where they were to complete the second half of their language studies. The cooler air in the hills was much appreciated.

Bags unpacked, Jean sat down to write to her family once again. She chuckled as she shared her latest bedbug encounter.

The girls settled in, and the second phase of language study began in earnest. One quiet evening, Jean penned another letter discussing family news and her activities:

> Today I went to the bazaar. I love to go even if I don't buy a thing. The stores are so fascinating even if they are not much to look at. The people are fascinating too, and so natural in their ways. I wish you could just, for a few days, see our people. I certainly never regret the day I came here. Sometimes the job seems bigger than I could ever do, and I know without Him I could do nothing, but I am doing all for Him, no matter if I give my life for Him; that would be so little. I shall never forget the fact that He changed my life and I know I will be with Him forever. I love His people, both here in India and in our country. Life is worthwhile when we live it for Him. And when things come up that trouble us, there is a peace that makes the troubles minor…

Outside, the rains of India poured down, and inside the girls poured over their studies, sometimes reading aloud from their books. In June, Jean, along with sixteen other missionaries, wrote the second part of the exams.

"I am so happy to be done with them," Jean announced to Ruth as they walked back to the bungalow. "I just pray I'll be truly proficient in the days ahead."

Ruth laughed. "You're not the only one."

After a brief break, the group returned to Basim. Jean had planted a flower and vegetable garden outside their home in the complex, and rejoiced to see the fruit of her labours.

Some foods were scarce, flour and potatoes among them. Doctor Speicher wrote to the mission to ask if they could send white flour once a month, and Jean wrote home asking for packets of Jell-o and dried fruit.

On the Sunday following their return, Jean cycled to church, as usual. She preferred this mode of transport, rather than waiting for the car or the jeep.

"Good morning, Bhagiai," she called to one of her student nurses.

"Good morning, Sister Darling." Bhagiai beamed. "This is the day the Lord has made, isn't it."

"Yes, indeed." Jean marveled as she reflected on this little nurse's faith. She recalled the elders of the village going to the girl's parents to express their concern about Bhagiai's situation. The young nurse had a husband who beat her frequently, and the men had advised the parents to take her back into their home. This had been done, but when the husband became desperately ill she had gone back into the home to nurse him, and before he died she led him to the Lord. Eventually, Bhagiai married one of the Indian pastors. *What a Savior,* Jean thought.

They entered the church together, greeting people as they did. The Indian pastors conducted the services, and some of the women taught Sunday school. Jean sat on the floor as was the custom. The events that followed prompted another letter home.

Well, I have had one more interesting and new experience. It was at church this morning. I have had everything bite me, from bedbugs to I don't know what, but about five minutes after we sat on the floor for Sunday school, I was alive with lice! There were hundreds of them crawling all over my sari and I was picking them off my face.

Needless to say, Jean and Agnes, one of the missionaries who had also been targeted, grabbed their bikes. They pedaled furiously back to the bungalow amid shrieks and laughter as they slapped the pests from their bodies while trying to keep the bikes on course. Rushing into the bungalow, they shook liberal amounts of DDT powder over themselves, until the offending critters succumbed. They then bathed, sprinkled more powder in their hair, and wrapped towels tightly around their heads.

"That should take care of any who escaped into our heads," Jean announced. "We could keep the towels on for a while. Let's have a tea first."

A little breathless and amid bursts of laughter, they sat at the kitchen table and did just that.

"We have council meeting next week," Agnes said.

"Yes. I'm not slated to attend that one," Jean remarked. "Just as well. We are so busy in the hospital. You know the activities of missionaries never cease, do they. We have our teachers at the Bible School headed up by the Andersons, then there's the evangelists, administrators and educators. Those ministering in the villages and some working at the hospital. Brother Prescott Beal is a wonderful leader, isn't he? His enthusiasm is so contagious."

"You can say that again."

Their adventure over and tea done, they set to and washed their hair.

The months passed by and Christmas came soon enough. With her student nurses, Jean again prepared for the festive season as 1947 came to a close.

Missionary Travels
(An ode to bed parasites)

I want to cheer you up dear folk and tell you something bright,
That millions of our Hindustan aren't starving much tonight.
The bedding roll was all prepared and then I crawled inside
To snuggle in and go to sleep, but soon, "What's that?" I cried.
"We can't afford to starve all night, we're out for blood that's red.
We thought you wouldn't mind a bit, if we came here to beg."
"It isn't fair, you did not ask, if you could feast tonight.
You just brought your swords along and poked me left and right."
"But this is why we marched right on," they answered with a blow.
"My mom, my pop, my sis, and son, are hungry don't you know?"
"Now I must kill you off right quick, the reason I will give;
Old maidens like to be alone, in peacefulness to live."
Just see my arms and legs and feet all bitten up and sore;
And see my pillow, sheets and clothes, all stained from this great war."
"I'll move my bedroll off the bench and sleep down on the floor.
Then you'll be sad, I tell you now, 'cause you'll all starve the more."
"But then we'll go with you," they cried. "We tell you we're your
friend,
And when you go to sleep once more, we'll come and camp again."
"Well I give up, you've won tonight, for now my sleep has gone,
But I'll sit up and pen this ode and catch you as you come."
"Yes, you're right smart. You sneak along, but see you cannot win.
Instead of being big and fat, your figures still are slim."
"It's five o'clock, I'll leave you now—the night has gone at last.
Once more I hope and pray to God, that nights with you are past."
Jean Darling, 1947

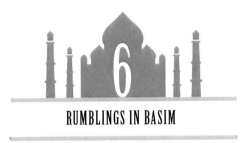

6

RUMBLINGS IN BASIM

Halfway through January, 1948, Jean wrote home once more:

> …We had a wonderful camp meeting. I came home tired out, of course. It takes a lot of strength to really pray, and we stayed up late at night and got up early in the morning. However, it was wonderful—many young people got saved…I had been praying for a long, long time. I was thrilled.

In the quiet of the early morning, Jean watched the nursing students file into the courtyard. They sat down on the mats under a tree and bowed their heads in prayer, asking God to help them with their studies and their Christian walk. They prayed especially for the ones who would be writing their exams that week. Jean had prepared the exam papers, and with a grateful heart she thanked God for the progress made. A second group of students would enter the nurses' training program later in the year.

Exams over, Jean took a break. Sister Geraldine Chappell, who mostly looked after dispensary, and Doctor Evelyn Witthoff, both of whom had recovered from internment by the Japanese during World War II, oversaw the nurses and patient care while Jean went on a field trip with fellow missionaries.

They set off in two jeeps. Paula and Bronell Greer and Jean in one, Leslie Fitzlan, Mr. Bhuphal, Doctor Barde, and a cook in the other. The group set up camp and lived in tents. Each day, they visited people and churches in the surrounding villages and shared the good news of the gospel.

"We have to visit the Ajanta Caves while we are here," Doctor Barde announced.

"Is there something special about them?" Jean asked.

Doctor Barde's eyes twinkled. "Centuries ago, in fact, in the first and second century BC, Buddhist monks claimed a horseshoe-shaped cliff, high in the mountainside along the Waghora River. They carved out monasteries and hallways, intricate carvings and prayer rooms, as well as a giant Buddha. Not only that, you will see murals on some of the walls. It is believed they lived there for nine centuries. No one knows when the caves were vacated, but they were discovered in 1819, by a British explorer on a tiger hunt, or I guess you could say rediscovered."

Jean and her companions were not disappointed. The spectacular caves had them taking numerous photos. During their trek back, they came across a heap of bones, the remains of men who had died in one of the many skirmishes and fights. India was awash with conflict and no area escaped some catastrophe.

"Do you suppose we could take some of these bones for my nursing classes?" Jean said.

Paula looked hard at Jean. "Are you serious?"

"Yes, teaching materials are scarce and a real skeleton would be a bonus."

"I don't see why not," Doctor Barde said.

And with that, he and the other men in the party collected a bag of bones! When Jean got back to the hospital, she used them in her anatomy classes.

In April, Jean and Ruth, due for physical checkups, travelled to Bombay, where the intense heat forced them to change clothes several times in a day. The hot dry season dictated the necessity for the closing of the hospital for a few weeks, due to a shortage of water.

The next month, the missionaries attended a Christian conference in Kodaikanal, a beautiful spot in the hills of southern India 1,500 miles from Basim. Attendees came from several denominations. Jean eagerly participated in a workshop on photography and film. She hoped eventually to procure a projector, not only to film the sights of India, but to obtain educational film from the National Indian Board for her nursing classes. Remaining in Kodaikanal through June, Jean along with others visited the Temple of Madura; of it, she wrote:

> …It was very hot, 103 degrees…by 4:00pm we were all exhausted—our eyes sunken, our faces flushed until we scared each other. We went all through the temple. We had to walk around in our stocking feet, because it was sacred ground… There were merchants by the dozen buying and selling—no wonder Jesus drove them out. Anything that could be had in India was there for sale. There were 1,000 pillars and on every pillar an idol of a human or an animal. Men and women came before them, put their hands up to their faces, and made requests. Some lay prostrate before the gods…there were idols all over the place. Heathenism is a terrible thing; one can hardly describe what it is like.
>
> Then we came back Tuesday, glad to get out of the heat. We stayed at the mission hospital overnight, and I enjoyed seeing it and getting ideas.
>
> My holiday is almost gone and I can hardly wait to get back to work. I guess I wasn't made for long rests. I go back to Basim on June 25, and our hospital will open July 1. In August, a new class of nurses will come in…

The return journey was long and arduous, with challenges to boot. With the rumblings of a showdown in Hyderabad State, people moved in droves from one place to another, trying to escape conflict and a place to settle. At the railway station, soldiers and police were everywhere. Men of less-than-noble character stole from passengers, and Jean did not escape unscathed. A thief broke into her compartment in the train by forcing a window open and then reached in and stole her shopping bag with much-needed supplies she had purchased for the hospital. Upon her arrival home, she penned yet another letter to her family.

...Doctor Speicher is keeping house, so she is making cookies now. It is a relief not to have the extra work, even though I enjoy keeping house so much. I have been getting all the equipment ready for the hospital, for in the rainy season we need a lot more linens for they do not dry as fast. On August 1, we take in a new class. I do not know how many yet...I have to get my courses outlined both for Doctor Speicher and I to teach them, so will be kept busy for a while. I hope to get in some Marathi study, too...

As Jean sealed her letter, Kissen knocked on the bungalow door.

"Good morning, Sister," he said with a smile. "I am ready to drive you."

"Just coming, Kissen." Jean grabbed her bag. For a few weeks, on Wednesday mornings, she had been assigned to go to the missionaries' boarding school some seventy miles away in Chikhli. New missionaries Cleve and Nita James were getting acclimatized to the work. Two hundred and fifty children boarded there, and Jean provided knowledge and support to them.

Jean knew her family waited for her letters, and with diligence wrote, giving them much insight into the life of a missionary, all of whom wore several hats. The rainy season had started in June and did not stop until September, although there were breaks during this period. As she typed her letter of July 24, she looked up for a moment and stared out of her window at the rain. Tapping away at the keys, she wrote:

…It has been raining all week, but at present has stopped. The weather is wonderful and good for sleeping at night. I like it to rain in the afternoon, for then the kids do not make a racket playing outside and I can sleep! Guess I'm getting to be more of an old maid. We have nine orphans just back of my door and window, so they make a noise along with the other compound children.

Saturday, Doctor S had to go to Chikhli to bring a boy back from the school…he is very sick with typhoid fever. We do not know if he will make it or not. She got back yesterday afternoon but was very tired, so she let me deliver a baby this afternoon. We have a lot of cases lately, and I'm glad, for it keeps the nurses in practice. Just now I have come from the hospital, after raiding (DDT) all the bathrooms and checking up on the linen, etc.

The patients go out to have a stool anywhere in the grass or anywhere they can find a clean space! But I have gotten after them so much that they are pretty good to go to the outside toilets now.

The mail is about to go, so I must close for this time. I was fixing flowers in the house and forgot to look at the time. I am going to plant seeds, as the gardener is getting the earth all fixed up. They should have been planted a long time ago, but we never got around to it and the seeds were not here. That is what I should like to have next year: some good seeds from home. If you send them by March, I would get them in time. All kinds of vegetable and flower seeds. Evelyn Whitthoff brought some with her last year and we had the best garden from those seeds.

Did I tell you I have a lady working in my room now to keep everything straight? She does my washing, cleans and dusts, waters my plants, mends my clothes, etc. I pay her four dollars a month. It is wonderful to come home and not have to do all those things. It always takes twice as long to get things done here. At the hospital it is the same, and one gets weary trying to get things done at the same speed as one does at home.

At home there is just the nursing to look after, but here we have to see they get all the privileges that will help them spiritually, too.

Three nurses hurried across the compound and down the lane to the church. Sister Darling had arranged for them to be at the 8:30 am revival meeting. The church was packed and an air of excitement filled the sanctuary. A missionary from the Alliance Church spoke powerfully morning and evening, encouraging all in their faith. Jean had slated the rest of the student body to attend the evening service.

A cool breeze stirred on an early September evening as Doctor Speicher, Mary Anderson and Jean walked along the lane.

"This is so refreshing," Jean said. "I love this time of year."

Doctor Speicher agreed. "Yes. It's nice to get a bit of a break." She stooped and picked a flower from a nearby bush. "The past week has been wonderful with all the preachers meetings."

Mary spoke. "I've heard excellent reports. People went away truly blessed."

"And we're being blessed with scads of babies," Jean interjected. "God has blessed us with good students, too, which reminds me, tomorrow I have to give out the weekly portions of grain and supplies to the nurses who are boarding, and to Kavitha for the orphans. I hope the sun comes out strong so I can sun and dry the grain. Funny how the sun kills the bugs. But I'm glad it does."

Doctor Speicher stopped and looked at her companions.

"We could be in for some tough times ahead if the Hyderabad situation isn't settled soon. The soldiers and police coming into the village are disturbing."

"Yes, and we're so close to the border," Jean said.

"That's right. Let's keep praying for a peaceful resolution."

But it was not to be.

Jean lay in her bed in the bungalow. What she and her friends hoped for had not come about, and her ears strained for the familiar sound, the low rumble, and then it came—heavy tanks moving stealthily into Basim. She prayed in silence, *Dear God, whatever is to come, protect us and help us to minister where needed.* The threat of war that had loomed over India now seemed a reality, and Basim, twelve miles from the border of Hyderabad, had become the conduit to launch an attack. The Hyderabad dispute had finally come to a head. Its ruler had appealed to the newly formed United Nations to settle the issue, and also to the British Labour Party and the king, but all to no avail.

An Indian army officer came to the hospital flanked by two others. "We are requesting that you vacate the premises," he said to Doctor Speicher. "We will need it for our injured."

"We will stay and we will take care of your wounded," Doctor Speicher told him.

"Well doctor, if you insist, but I cannot guarantee your safety."

"We will pray to our God," she said.

The official looked at her for a moment then turned on his heel and walked away.

Basim was in turmoil. The Indian Union Government and police had taken over the schools, the cotton gin, and the jail to house their own. Many of the villagers fled. Mary Anderson and her husband took the students from the Bible College away on a prolonged tour. Their bungalow became home to Indian officials.

One September morning, Jean and Doctor Speicher watched two officials coming across the hospital courtyard.

"Good morning, Doctor," one said. "We are sending eight wounded to you. They will arrive in the next fifteen minutes."

Jean felt a surge of excitement. *We will be caring for Hindus and Mohammedans,* she thought.

It seemed Doctor Speicher read her thoughts. "Let's pray God will become real to them all, Jean."

The two women watched as the injured, some on stretchers, came through the doors. Doctor Speicher quickly assessed each patient. They treated the most severely injured first, cleansing, suturing and bandaging gaping wounds. Jean took a moment to straighten up after working on a patient's leg; as she did, she heard frantic cries and looked up to see a woman with a young boy.

"They shot him in the head," she wailed.

"Over here. Put him on the cot."

The woman trembled as she laid the boy down. Jean gently removed the towel from the child's head. Blood and tissue stained the cloth, and part of his brain protruded from the gaping hole. Doctor Speicher hurried over and examined the child. She cleansed the wound and sutured the damaged dura mater back together.

"Best to apply a pressure bandage," she said to Jean. That done, the child settled.

The doctor, student nurses, Jean, and Christian helpers prayed constantly as they tended the sick. More patients were admitted with war wounds over the next couple of days.

On day twelve, Hyderabad ceded to the Indian government.

When army officials returned to the hospital to assess the status of the patients, they exclaimed amazement at the recovery of the injured. A small Indian helper looked at them and said softly, "It's because we pray for them."

The official stared in disbelief as the boy with the brain injury scooted across the room, laughing. A nurse called after him.

During this upheaval, news had filtered through to Doctor Speicher that once again an outbreak of bubonic plague had occurred in a village fifteen miles away. The evidence—a large number of flea-ridden rats, had been found dead in the area. Doctor Speicher turned to Jean.

"The villagers will have gone to the fields again. Whenever the plague occurs, that's what happens, as we well know. Our villagers were inoculated last time, so we'll pray they remain healthy. "

Amid these difficulties, the missionaries stayed focused on their work. Jean, ever faithful to keep her family informed, wrote:

September 28, 1948

These have been very busy days all right. Doctor Speicher was away and just came back today, in fact just now, so I had her work to do as well as my own. All the cases that came in during the war have to have their wounds dressed and it takes time. We had a baby born on Monday at four in the morning and another lady came in very ill who had her baby...I think we are getting an Indian doctor, so that will help…I am going to try and find an Indian graduate nurse when I go to Jubbulpore, so maybe I'll have some spare time, too. I do not want you to think that I do too much; I do not do half as much as I need to do, and would like to do. But we cannot work nearly so hard here and get by with it physically as we can at home.

I am feeling much better and can eat everything now. I am taking scads of vitamins and my hair has almost stopped falling out. It was terrific for a while after I came home from the hills. It did that the first year I was here until I only had half the hair I had at the beginning. Well enough of that blah.

Everything is getting settled down after the war. There are still some troubles in the little villages, I guess, but that, too, is being taken care of now. I sure appreciate the opportunity that we had to help, even if it was in a little way.

I will have to go to a convention in Yeotmal and will come back on the 17th, I believe. Then our missionaries' yearly council meeting is from the 26th–30th. So, you see, our time plans itself out for us.

Jean yawned and stretched. She typed a closing paragraph, telling her folks about the abundance of fruits and vegetables in the garden, and then headed to her room. She was ready for bed.

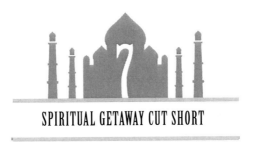

SPIRITUAL GETAWAY CUT SHORT

THE HALL BUSTLED WITH ACTIVITY. MISSIONARY NURSES AND INDIAN nurses greeted one another. Their conversations dwelt on the current issues of the day, as well as their respective hospitals' progress.

Jean had left Basim during the first week of October and travelled north to Jubbulpore, stopping on the way to visit the Missionary Alliance Mission. Then she had looked forward to the nurses' convention.

She was not disappointed. *It's wonderful,* she thought. *I'm really feasting on spiritual things as I never have since coming to India.*

Her reflections were interrupted when she heard her name being called from the front of the hall. "Jean Darling."

"Here," she waved to the speaker who held a telegram in her hand. Jean hurried to the front, anxious to know the content.

The speaker spoke to Jean, then addressed the nurses. "Doctor Speicher is very sick with malaria and dengue fever." Jean didn't wait to hear more; she hurried to her room, packed her belongings, and returned to Basim.

While Doctor Speicher recovered, Jean oversaw the general care of patients with the help of her student nurses and the workers. By the end of October, Doctor Speicher improved in time for Jean to attend the three-day annual council meeting, held at the Bible College. Of it, she wrote:

> October 16, 1948
> We had a wonderful council meeting this year. It lasted from Tuesday morning to Friday evening. The folks went home yesterday. There were nineteen of us and five children. The service Friday night lasted until 2:00 am, and none of us wanted to come home. It was surely a camp meeting and we enjoyed the blessings so much. We needed it, for unless we get filled up, we cannot give out to the people…

One afternoon, in a letter to her sister, Jean admonished her for being too concerned:

> November 11, 1948
> Grace, you make me feel silly, telling me I do too much, for really I do not. If I did what I would like to do, I would do five times as much. But it isn't how much work a person does, or even how clever a person is, but how he or she lives, and what one contributes to other lives by attitude and help. I heard someone say, one time, that he didn't think the Lord was interested in how much work we do, but in how we do it. Sometimes we get so busy we haven't time to put the emphasis on the value of lost souls, and that is more important than any amount of work one could ever do…

"Hello there." Jean smiled at Mary Anderson from the Bible School as she came into the bungalow.

"It's amazing how cold it gets inside, isn't it?" Mary said, as she checked a plate of cookies on the kitchen table. She looked at Jean.

"Sure, go ahead. I'll have one, too. Do you want a tea?"

"Give you three guesses," Mary said, as she turned on the tap. With the pot on the stove, she perched herself on the kitchen stool and munched on her cookie. "Can you believe it? Christmas is just around the corner again. The Bible students are so enthused. They are practicing Christmas carols, and plan to put on a nativity play."

"It's such a special time of year. I'm writing *Away in a Manger* in Marathi," Jean said. "I'm going to teach it to the children. We'll do a play as well. By the way, I'm looking forward to Thursdays, Mary. It will be great to be visiting in the village once a week. Three more months and Doctor Evelyn Witthoff will be on staff here. That will be such a help. She's been very busy running clinics in the villages. We'll all be able to have a day off. Did I tell you the new nurses wrote their exams last week, and they did well? I'm proud of them."

With a twinkle in her eye, Mary responded. "Yes, you did, and you've a right to be pleased. By the way, I noticed the vegetable garden doesn't look very good."

Jean pulled a face. "No. One little carrot showed up, and all we have are some tomatoes. We did have lettuce earlier in the year, and some celery. We used the celery to flavour our soups."

"Meat is scarce, isn't it," Mary said, "And I do not care for the goat meat, which is very expensive."

"I know. We eat canned meat nearly all the time, but have a variety so it's not too bad. There'll be food parcels coming any day now. I want to make candy, and I've ordered some walnuts from Bombay. I just hope they're not wormy."

Tea finished, Mary left and Jean went back to her typewriter. "Oh no," she announced to the empty room. The familiar sound of falling rain reached her ears. She went to the window and witnessed a downpour. The rainy season was officially over, and here in the middle of November it started again. It rained all night. Jean lay in bed praying for the cotton and crop-growers. Her next letter home told the sad story.

November 21, 1948

Even though the rainy season is over, this last week it has rained every night. The crops are ruined. The Javari—they ground it to make bread—and the cotton crops were just ready to harvest; there has been so much loss. Poor people, for at the very best they have very little. They grow three crops a year. I guess that is why the ground peters out so, for they never use fertilizer…It is raining now, so I am undressed, ready for bed. It is only 7:00 pm. The days are so short now, and I do not like it. It gets dark around 5:30–6:00 pm and light at 6:00 am…

"My family asked after you in their last letter." Jean sat across the table from Doctor Speicher. They were enjoying a curry made by their Indian cook.

"I hope you told them I'm all better," Doctor Speicher said, as she spooned up another mouthful.

"I did. This curry is so good. I love the taste of all the spices." Jean looked at her companion. "Thinking of all things good puts me in mind of an incident this morning. But maybe I shouldn't tell you while we're eating."

"I'm sure I can stomach it."

"This afternoon, after a baby was delivered, the sweeper woman put the placenta outside to dispose of it, but before she could, a crow flew down and took off with it. The forceps were still attached. The poor nurse was so upset about losing those forceps."

Both women started to laugh, and couldn't stop.

"Oh how funny," Doctor Speicher chortled, wiping tears from her eyes. "Well, I guess that's God taking care of that bird's needs."

"I suppose," Jean said, regaining her composure. "On another note, I wonder if Mr. Beals made it to my family's home or not. I know if he did they would enjoy him. He is a wonderful missionary and a wonderful preacher, isn't he?"

"How right you are. Samuelrao will be back with us soon. He's another great man of God. He was to leave by plane November 22nd, and to arrive in Bombay December 8th."

"I can hardly wait until he comes," Jean said. "I look forward to hearing of his experiences and impressions of the Western world. It will be a change and an adjustment to work among his own people again."

The meal finished, Jean announced she would clear up and get ready for bed. "I'll be going with Mary to minister in the village tomorrow," she said. "But right now I must fill my hot water bottle. The temperature changes are so drastic. I froze at night until I started using a hot water bottle."

"It's a damp, penetrating type of cold," Doctor Speicher said. "Yet the sun during the day is so warm. Don't forget, we've planned a getaway on Saturday. A picnic is a lovely idea. We'll have fellowship with the Lees and the Andersons. The men can build a fire if it gets too cold."

Singing softly as she washed up dishes, Jean thought about the class she had conducted with the nursing students that afternoon. It had gone well and the students were always so attentive. Chores finished, she reclined in her armchair and reflected on her missionary life thus far, then she took up her journal and smiled as she read a couple of poems she had written earlier.

A Conversation with God
I do not know why my work is here,
But God did send me, this much is clear.
Few times discouraged, to pastures green,
I wandered afar. Much have I seen.

But then I come back, the truth to face.
I know in my heart, this is my place.
It is the dark clouds, the sleet, the rain,
The storm and the gale that causes pain.

But in the distress, myself I see.
It is not from the sleet or the rain, but me.
So tender but firm, the Master says,
"The cloud for a while will hide bright rays,

But wait for the sun; it will not be long,
For sunshine with rain will make you strong."
So now there's no place I'd rather be
Than here in Basim where he sent me.
Jean Darling

Tonight the year of forty nine, into the yesterdays,
Will cross the mighty bridge of time. And there will rest always.
It causes me to look behind, review this year each day,
As I have tried to walk with Him, along the narrow way.

One day God came and whispered low, "I have a work for you."
I understood not what He meant, but pledged that work to do.
Then as He opened up His will and touched my blinded eyes
Anew, I caught a glimpse of those, who need revival fires.

And then he said so soft and clear, "Wait by faith on Me,
And bridge the gap till they come in. This is My work for thee."
Then when, by grace, my all I gave to Him for this great task.
My heart had only one request, "Thy strength each day I ask."

I felt so small, to Him I went and cried on bended knee,
"To do thy will in Hindustan, I must be more like thee."
He looked down from His heavenly home. My heart the Christ could
see;
His face, as I had never known, with love shone down on me.

He asked, "You're sure you wish to tread this weary way with Me?
And do you wish to pay the price, so great to Christ-like be?"
Then I out stretched my hand to Him. He took it in His own,
And filled my heart with peace, and love, that I had never known.
Jean Darling, 1949

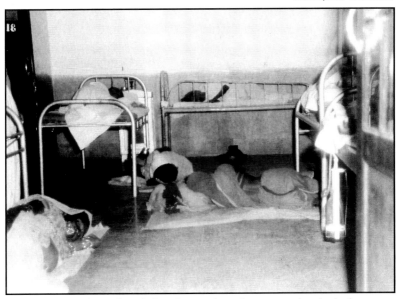

Medical ward with family members sleeping under the bed.

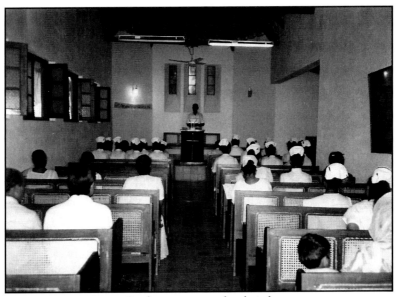

Student nurses in the chapel.

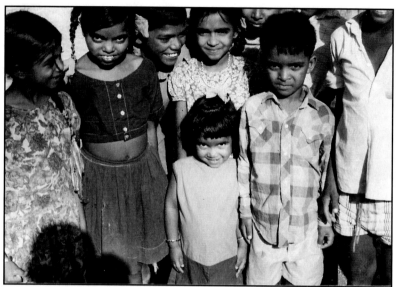

The little girl in the center later graduated from the nursing school.

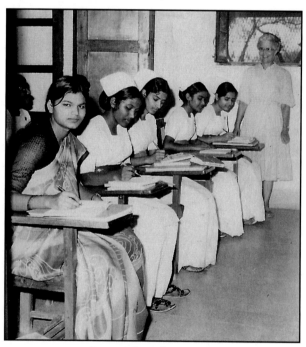

Jean with student nurses.

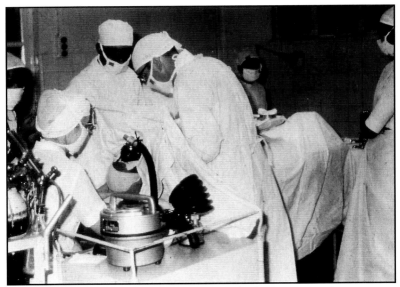

Jean assisting doctors in surgery and administering ether.

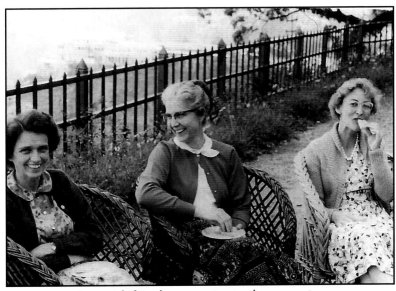

Jean with friends on vacation in the mountains.

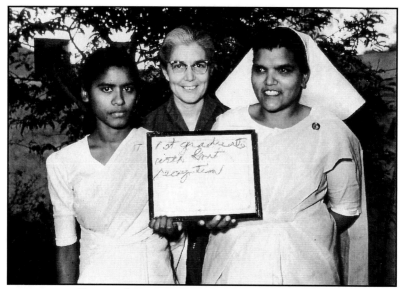

First graduate to receive government recognition.

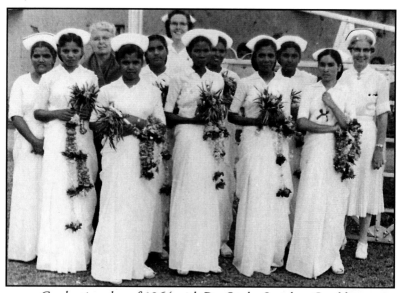

Graduating class of 1964 with Dr. Orpha Speicher, Geraldine and Jean in the back row.

At right:
Jean in her sari, 1975.

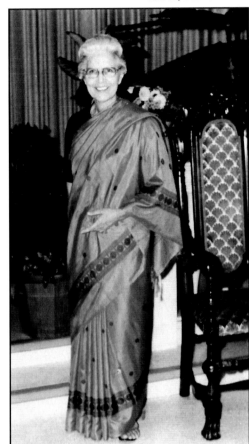

Below:
Golden Jubilee RMH,
1988. From left to right,
Jean with Carolyn Myatt
and Dr. Orpha Speicher.

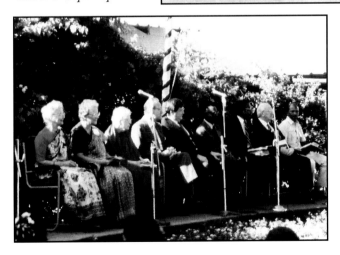

63

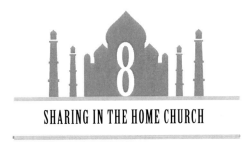

8

SHARING IN THE HOME CHURCH

J EAN PICKED UP A SMALL VASE FROM AN ASSORTMENT OF GIFTS SHE had on the kitchen table. She handed it to Mary, who sat wrapping each item with care in tissue paper.

"Can you believe it," Jean said, "five years have gone already. I have mixed feelings about going home to Canada. But I'll be happy to see my family."

"You will be so busy with deputation and visiting churches, telling people about your adventures in India and your beloved Basim, you will feel like you're still here," Mary said.

"I suppose." Jean brushed away a tear.

"You need a hug," Mary announced. She stood and delivered a big one to her friend. "Don't forget, you're coming back."

"That's right." Jean, energized by her own response, left Mary to finish wrapping the gifts and went into her bedroom. There she methodically sorted out the clothes she needed to pack.

"How you doing?" Mary stood in the doorway. "Your gifts are all wrapped."

"Thanks, my friend. I'll finish deciding what to take. I have to think cold and snow to start with. Mind you it's February now, and by March, Canada could be into thawing mode. But in any event, I have to write to Mom and let her know my route home."

"Okay. I'll get back to the college. See you later."

Jean thanked her, finished sorting, and placed some of her clothes in the case. *I might be changing my mind on some of this before I leave,* she thought.

She left Basim on March 3.

> March 10, 1951, onboard SS Chusan, PO Lines
> Dear Mom,
>
> It seems like a dream that I am on my way home. The ship is beautiful, with about 1,000 passengers. I have a cabin all to myself. I go up on deck a lot and enjoy the sea breezes. I couldn't describe it now, but will when I get home. There is nothing more thrilling than a sea voyage and I love every minute of it. There are just three Canadians and two Americans on board; all the rest are British, Chinese and Indian. But all are very interesting characters. The food is delicious. For each place-setting there are five knives, five forks and two or three spoons. There are so many courses, one could not possibly eat them all. We stop at Aden tomorrow, so will get off and see what there is to buy...

Jean went on to describe a variety of activities offered to the passengers, then closed her letter:

> Must go now. Church is at 10:00 am. It seems strange to have church onboard. Will write from England.

She stood on the deck in the blustery March wind, shading her eyes in an effort to see the missionary couple who were to meet her, but there were just too many people. She'd have to wait until they disembarked. They saw her first and waved enthusiastically, calling her name.

A whirlwind year of deputation began for Jean. For the first two weeks, she spoke to congregations in England and then Scotland. She told of her life and the work God had called her to do in India. She shared many stories of God's grace with her eager listeners. Jean then sailed home to Canada.

In her own church, London First Church of the Nazarene, she shared one incident when eight people from the Baptist mission a hundred miles away from Basim brought a child to the hospital late one night. The boy had been bitten by a rabid dog.

Looking out at the congregation, she said, "The group had sent a telegram, but they arrived before it did. The night watchman banged on our bungalow door, waking me and Doctor Speicher from a deep sleep. We pulled on gowns and hurried over to the outpatients'. The child had been given a vaccine, the parents said, but he still exhibited signs of rabies.

"While Doctor Speicher examined and treated the boy, I wondered what refreshments I could offer the family. A thought popped into my head," Jean said, as she scanned the congregation. "A cup of cold water in my name, and that's what I offered them. With Doctor Speicher's help, we made sleeping arrangements for the group. The Lord led me to pray with the mother, and together we committed the child into the loving care of the Father. The next morning, the mother told me that after the prayer, the child became quiet and slept the rest of the night."

Smiling, Jean told her audience a happy and grateful family returned home with a boy well on the way to recovery.

"Let me tell you about Bhakshibai," Jean said, as the applause and praise died down. "Bhakshibai's husband was a patient in the hospital. His private room was near the chapel. All patients who were able, and their relatives, were welcome to attend the morning chapel service. This little lady would come and sit on the floor just inside the chapel. One day she noticed a picture of Jesus surrounded by children, and close to Him a little Indian girl in a sari. Bhakshibai marveled at the picture. It amazed her that Jesus had an Indian girl close to Him—a girl who received no recognition in her own culture." Jean paused and looked around the packed church. "Can you guess what happened?"

"She gave her heart to the Lord," a lady called out.

"That's right. Bhakshibai became a joyful Christian and very dear to the missionaries. When family members were prescribed medications, she would administer them personally, saying, 'I give you this medicine in the name of Jesus.'"

So, for a year, Jean travelled and shared, stirring up the hearts of young and old alike with her stories of India.

Thy Hand

Thy hand, Oh Lord, so beautiful, so pure,
so full of grace and yet so strong and sure,
Is still outstretched to all with love untold.
And bleeding, points the way into the fold.
Thy healing hand, so blessed sought in prayer,
that touched blinded eyes, the heart of care,
Is waiting ever near to cleanse, to bless,
that man may know and share thy holiness.
Thy mighty hand, that turned the water into wine,
that fed the multitudes with bread divine,
Still pens the word, Ask much of Me,
that mountains be removed into the sea.
Thy tender gentle hand to prune the vine,
to break and mold the clay, and gold refine,
Is kind, yet firm, so true and keen,
that in each heart Thine image may be seen.
Thy faithful hand that calls and sends with care
each messenger Thy Light and love to bear
Though' scarred, will ne'er forsake,
will safely guide each step till dawn doth break.
Jean Darling, 1951

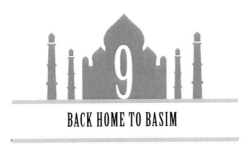

9

BACK HOME TO BASIM

"THE MODES OF TRAVEL I'VE EXPERIENCED ARE VARIED INDEED." Jean lay on her bed with her hands tucked under her head.

"We've got that to look forward to," Esther Howard said, as she perched on the end of the bed, hugging her knees to her chest.

"And it's good to know God is in charge and will direct us," Mary Harper added.

Jean's companions, both nurses from America, were setting out on their first missionary journey. The steady throbbing of the ship's engines and the gentle swell of the sea caused Jean to close her eyes.

It was August, 1952. They had pulled out of New York Harbour some three hours previous, aboard the MS Hoegh Trader, a Norwegian cargo ship. The crew were all Norwegian, with Indian servants who spoke Marathi.

The ringing of the dinner bell made her jump up. Apart from three priests, Jean and her two fellow travelers were the only passengers. "I feel sorry for those priests," Jean said, as they made their way to the dining room. "They go to the country of their calling for life. Never going home on furlough."

"I don't think I could stand that," Mary said, sighing.

The voyage passed well enough. In spite of their limited English, the crew were friendly. They taught the girls to play quoits, a simple game, where rings made of rope were tossed at a certain spot and marks were awarded accordingly. Sometimes they engaged in cards and dominoes. Mary played her accordion and the three women sung praises to God, their voices blending in harmony.

They took their meals at the captain's table. The captain showed surprise when the girls refused the wine offered. He told them his previous passengers had drinking parties every night.

The ship sailed on across the Atlantic Ocean and through the Straits of Gibraltar, with stops in Port Sudan, reaching Beirut in the fall.

On September 10, Jean's heart soared as she stepped onto Indian soil again. Geraldine Chappell met the girls in Bombay, where they boarded a train for Akola.

"This is where you get off," Jean announced to Esther and Mary as the train pulled into Malkapur. Hugs and goodbyes were said as they alighted, for they were to go on to Buldana and from there to language school.

"It's so good to see you," Geraldine said, as the train pulled out of the station.

"I'm happy to be back, my friend," Jean said, smiling. She shared some of her activities over the past year during the rest of the journey. Arriving at Akola Station, Jean peered out of the window to see Doctor Speicher on the platform, with Doctor Cox and his son Ira Lee. Doctor Cox was to join the staff at the hospital. Greetings exchanged, they made their way to Basim.

After a couple of days, Jean pulled out her typewriter. She had to get a letter sent to her family.

September 19, 1952

We arrived in Bombay last Friday afternoon. It was a job to get our freight onto the train. Geraldine stayed over and brought it later. Saturday, we went shopping. I got the vegetables and had lots of fun bargaining...you have a dull time shopping in comparison to us. It was wonderful to rattle away in Marathi, and it seemed I'd never been away from India. I have everything unpacked and am trying to get settled. Yesterday, the nurses had a welcome service for Doctor & Mrs. Cox, and me. They gave us garlands. Then we made rounds and showed them the hospital. On my way home from Akola, the nurses had garlands for me and sang a welcome song, so I feel I've been welcomed plenty.

Jean had purchased a skeleton for her anatomy classes, and a large dummy for practical nursing instructions. She wrote:

You should have seen the Indian people when they opened the box with the skeleton in it. Their eyes were as big as saucers... and then the big doll in a box frightened them, too. Everybody was anxious to see, and we laughed until our sides were sore.

I think I shall sell my organ to Alberta Fletcher, for she does not have one and she has charge of the children in Mahableshwar. Doctor Speicher's is the same as mine and it has a rich, beautiful tone. I hate to let mine go, but will be able to play hers any time.

The missionary council meeting is next week and will be held in Basim, so I shall see all the missionaries then.

I must write to some folks at home when I get settled into the work. Geraldine is trying to get ready to go home, and with all the excitement one does not feel like settling down to anything...

Her letter finished, she hurried over to the hospital. In consult with Doctor Speicher, they had decided a young child in the hospital needed further assessment, and Jean would take the child to the Cancer Hospital in Bombay.

The train chugged along; Jean hugged the little orphan girl and allayed the child's fears. "Look at the cows, Aaruni. So many, aren't there."

The girl nodded. "Many cows," she said, her little face lighting up.

"Yes, and we'll see them all when we come home."

The child had a mole on her scalp, and the possibility it might be cancerous necessitated the appointment. The long trip took three nights of travel on the train there and back, but at the end of it all, the mole proved to be non-malignant.

Jean walked across the courtyard with Aaruni and deposited her small charge back into the orphanage, where the children greeted her with much chatter.

When Jean checked in at the hospital, Geraldine told her all was well. "Doctor and Mrs. Cox will soon be off to language school," she said.

"It is a long business now," Jean observed. "Two whole years before they'll be ready to join us. Well, I want to write to the family and bring them up to date."

She returned to her room and soon the steady click of the typewriter occupied her time.

October 6, 1952

Here it is Monday and I've been trying since Friday to write to you. The same people work at the hospital as before, except there is one new man and also a lab technician, as well as some new student nurses. Doctor Cox has been down, but in a couple of weeks, he and his wife go off to language school. In the meantime, we shall try to raise our standards and get ready to change the hospital from women and children to a general hospital. There will be a lot of change and a lot of headaches, too, but that's to be expected.

Geraldine is starting to pack now, and getting ready to go home—sailing on October 31. She is very thin, weighing only 124lbs and five feet, ten inches tall, so you can see she is just skin and bone. Tomorrow, the nurses are doing a special dinner for her and will give her a gift. I am looking forward to all the good food. They are preparing dudh curry, which is milk boiled down until it is quite thick, with spices, sugar, raisins, cocoanut and all kinds of rich things in it. We will have it with chapati (Indian flatbread), and after that we will have chicken curry— hot with spices. Zaibai, the nurses' cook, came Saturday to plan the meal, and then she went to the village to buy the supplies. She surely is a wonderful cook.

Doctor Speicher is having fever and not feeling well. We are a great bunch. It is so strange to see her go to bed as early as I do, for she always stayed up and read until the small wee hours, but she can't take it anymore.

We have septic tanks now, and have one bathroom completed. The other three will be done before long. It will be wonderful not to have the commodes and the sweepers coming three times a day…

"I'll have to call Doctor Vaze for this one." Jean stood at the bedside of a young mother who had given birth to a baby, but had not expelled the placenta. Her pulse was weak and irregular. Jean turned to the nurse standing beside her. "I'll be back in a minute."

Doctor Vaze arrived from the village and administered ether, then removed the placenta.

"It will be good when we can cross-match our patients' blood," Jean remarked to the doctor. "The poor mothers with their low hemoglobin make for a worrying time."

"How many deliveries have you had today?" the doctor asked.

"I've lost count. We have fifty-five inpatients, and you know what the outpatient is like."

Doctor Vaze glanced at her watch. "Well, Jean, I must be off. I hope you and the nurses have a quiet night. I'll see you in the morning."

Doctor Speicher was away and Jean, once again, over saw all patient care, apart from Doctor Vaze coming in for two and a half hours in the mornings.

"I'll be off, Nurse Bhagiai," Jean said to her senior night nurse. "After you've done medication rounds, you should have a quiet night. Our young mother is settled now and her vital signs are much improved. Tomorrow, I'll be away for prayer day. Nurse Aesha will be in charge." Jean rubbed her tummy. "I need to eat, and then I must get your salaries ready before I go to bed. Have a good night. God bless."

"Thank you, Sister," Bhagiai responded.

As Jean walked across the compound, her thoughts turned to the last letter she had received from home. Her brother Jack was ill. In response to the news, she had written:

…From the beginning, God has done much through the suffering of His people, for it is then, more than any other time, we are conscious of our helplessness and our need of Him. He will give strength to go through trials. I hope it is not cancer, but if it is we need not go to pieces, but hold on and believe for God to have His way and to work it out for our good. I have prayed and I know you have been praying, too…

"Bless my family, Lord, and be with Jack," Jean whispered as she entered the bungalow.

"I submit him to your care."

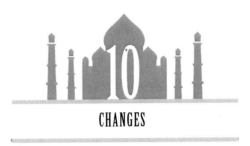

10

CHANGES

"HELLO, ESTHER. HOW GOES IT?" JEAN STOOD IN THE DOORWAY of her old office. Esther Howard had assumed Jean's role as Nurse Manager of the Nursing School.

"Hello there." Esther looked up from the papers she was scrutinizing. "I just finished checking the list of new applicants. It's so wonderful to have our students passing exams and moving into senior positions on the wards. And here you are, our Nursing Superintendent, and me in your old shoes."

"Look what the Lord has done," Jean said. "The fact that we are a recognized school by the Indian Board of Nursing is so gratifying. Any concerns, Esther?"

"None. I'll let you know if I need help. How are you feeling?"

"I'm on treatment round three for my malaria, and don't feel like skipping the rope yet. But it will pass," she said with a smile.

As Jean made her way back to the office, she felt the familiar chills of the disease coming on. "Oh no," she mumbled. She made her way to her room, where she would have to stay until it passed.

Jean lay on her bed covered in blankets and thought about a train journey she had taken to Bombay once, with heat so intense she had soaked towels in cold water and hung them in the train window. Her clothes had already been soaked in perspiration, so it made no difference, and the wet towels flapping on her as the train chugged along had brought some relief.

Now here she was, shivering. She managed a smile as she thought about the extreme temperatures in India. *But I wouldn't have it any other way,* she thought. *Thank you, Lord, for your guidance and protection,* she silently prayed.

Soon the chills subsided and she was ready to resume her work. She made herself tea and then headed for her office. On the way, she felt a surge of satisfaction. Doctor Evelyn Whittoff now worked at the hospital, as well as continuing basic health care classes to the women in the villages.

In 1955, a brief respite from work allowed Jean a vacation in Calcutta.

December 18, 1955

Mary Harper and I have had a wonderful trip. I did not think I would have enough money, since I felt I should give money for a seminary for young Indian men. I gave, but in gifts I received twice as much as I had given, so it has been an extra blessing.

We arrived in Darjeeling on December 14. It was very cold, and we piled on as many clothes as we could. On the way up the mountain, we travelled on the narrowest train in the world, just two feet wide. It looked like a big toy train…when we went down the mountain, the snow was beautiful and we feasted on that beauty for two days. We saw parts of Mount Everest…We visited the museum where all Sherpa Tenzing's climbing outfits are kept…

Missionaries continued to arrive in India. A great company of witnesses called to spread the good news—some to teach, some to administer, some to preach, and so on. The work moved forward, with teams visiting the villages, teaching the nationals and handing over more of the work to their Indian brothers and sisters. Each time the missionaries returned from furlough, the Indians held welcoming services for them, proving the power of God's love.

In the spring of 1959, Jean once again took leave of her beloved India, returning home to Canada, where she shared with many congregations her work in the field.

Upon her return, she considered the increase in nursing students and the many babies delivered at the hospital. An idea was forming in her mind, and she called Esther into her office and shared it with her.

Esther looked intently at Jean. "I really think it's an excellent idea. You'd be able to teach the course."

"Not only that, Doctor Speicher's been the only one teaching midwifery, and now with her away and facing cancer surgery, I can fill in the gap." Jean picked up the application form on her desk. It was from the midwifery school in the Bombay Hospital. "I'll apply for funding. I could be certified before the year is out."

After applying to take the course, she received the go-ahead, and was a certified midwife within six months. She returned from the hospital in Bombay and added teaching the midwifery course to her many roles.

One of the nationals, who, under Jean's supervision, was being schooled to step into the role of nursing superintendent, ably carried on with the work while Jean was away, and eventually became the nursing superintendent. A great achievement for Jean, for the missionary's goal was always to train and hand over to nationals.

The year of 1962 ended in tragedy for the missionary community. Jean sat at her desk and penned the events from her perspective:

I was with Bill & Lenora Pease in Chikhli for a few days in December. The morning of December 15, I made rounds of the girls' dorms with Lenora and shared her challenges. Then, while Lenora prepared goodies for a Christmas tea party for one or two classes of boys and girls, I went to my room. A great burden came upon me, but I didn't know for whom or what. I walked the floor and prayed until lunchtime.

After lunch, the Peases were preparing for another tea party. I sat down at the organ and played the hymn, *I'll go Where You Want Me to Go, Dear Lord.* Over and over again I sang that day; the Holy Spirit was present. I thought this must be for Lenora, but it puzzled me.

After the tea party, I enjoyed tea with Lenora and then prepared to take the bus back to Basim. Lenora begged me to stay overnight, but I was to be on duty at the hospital the next day. So I went home.

Between 10:00 & 11:00 pm, a phone call came through the post office that Lori Pease and David Greer had drowned. I packed some supplies of canned meats, powdered milk, eggs, bread, etc. and we—I don't remember who went with me in that car—drove to Chikhli. I learned that while Reverend Pease and his wife were holding evangelistic meetings in a village, their son Lori and his friend David had gone hunting birds. The birds fell on what appeared to be an island in a big pond. They went out to get the birds, and David got caught in the tall reeds. Lori tried to help him.

The next morning, the men went to find the boys. There was no island, just tall reeds. Cleve James had built a cover for his trailer, which he used for a boat, and they used that to bring the boys to shore. It took time for the police to release the bodies. While the men were gone, the ladies went to purchase saris for Lenora and Paula to wear to the funeral that afternoon.

I stayed in the bungalow, in case people came and needed food. I walked around the bungalow from one room to another. All of a sudden, the bungalow was filled with music and what seemed to be a thousand choirs singing praises because two boys had come home. I strained to hear more, but I could not understand the words. The doors were closed, because it was cold weather. I tried to find out where the music was coming from, but there were no radios on or any instruments. The choir kept singing and I kept walking, shocked by the beautiful music. It had to be angels singing. When some of the Indian people realized I was alone, they came to be with me and then the music stopped.

That afternoon, the funeral was held in the church. Lori was in a coffin made by the men. It was covered with a white cloth, with a cross on the lid. David was on the other side. The glory of the Lord came down as Mr. McKay gave a message.

After the funeral, a lady said, "You have taught us how to mourn."

Geraldine Chappell stayed with the Greers, and I stayed with the Peases for several days.

It was interesting that every time we met for prayer days, the glory of the Lord came upon us with a spirit of praise.

On a quiet afternoon in 1963, Jean opened a letter from her mother. Sitting on the side of her bed, she absorbed the news. Her father had passed away.

"Did he know you, Lord?" she asked out loud. "Oh, God, I pray he did."

Not long after that, she received a letter from a Mr. Sash and, elated, she read the contents. Then she wrote to her mother and siblings:

…I had a beautiful letter from Mr. Sash, telling how he led Dad to the Lord. He said the first step was when he (Dad) sent word to the church to pray for him and that he was praying for them. Then the next time, he said he had not been what he should have been, and after that Dad told him that he had asked Jesus to forgive his sins and he acknowledged Jesus as his Saviour.

Mr. Sash said that God worked in Dad's heart far above any way we could ask or think…

"I know whom I have believed," Jean sang as she walked across the compound to the hospital. "And I believe for Doctor Speicher," she said, as she pushed open the hospital door and walked in. "Hello, Norma. How you doing?"

"Good, thank you, Sister. I took a look around the wards. I'm meeting Esther in her office now." Norma Weiss was newly arrived from Canada and would be off to language school in two weeks. But Jean had suggested she familiarize herself with the hospital as much as possible before departing.

Jean cast a quick eye around the wards. Nurses were busy tending to the patients, and she acknowledged one or two as she did her rounds. Her mind turned to a request she had received from The United Church of Canada Hospital in Indore, a town north of Basim. Would she consider teaching some post-graduate nursing courses at their hospital? All was well at Reynolds Memorial, with a good and capable staff.

After council meeting, it was agreed Jean should go. For two months, from January to February 1965, she taught a body of student nurses in Indore. As well, she sat on the Executive Board of Nursing along with her peers from Christian hospitals in the district.

A significant event took place in Chikhli in December 1967. All the missionaries from the district attended a memorial service for Lori Pease and David Greer. A new chapel and library had been built onto the existing building in memory of the two friends. The money had been donated by Calgary First, the Peases' home church. The new additions were dedicated, and a prayer day followed.

The event brought peace to Jean and her contemporaries.

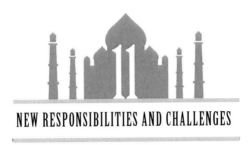

NEW RESPONSIBILITIES AND CHALLENGES

MEMBERS OF COUNCIL SAT AROUND THE TABLE IN THE BUNGALOW at Reynolds Memorial Hospital to view their options. The Indian Government had ruled that no more missionaries could come to India. But those working in the country would be allowed to return after furloughs.

Reverend Beals addressed the group. "We have to recognize our numbers will dwindle as people retire. But for now, let's look at the gifts we have and consider how best to utilize them. We do have four in language school right now, but they won't be ready to join us for another eighteen months."

Doctor Speicher, back from her time away after surgery, spoke. "The Peases are going on furlough. We need an administrator for the school in Chikhli. There are one hundred and fifty boarders and seventy-five day students, and without a doubt the numbers are going to grow."

Jean nodded and raised an eyebrow as Doctor Speicher looked at her. "Jean, you have proved you have a great head for figures, for leadership, and management. Would you consider taking up the reins at the school?"

Reverend Beals inclined his head and waited.

"Yes, of course," Jean said. "Esther has a good handle on hospital administration, as well as the training school, and we have some excellent nurses in senior positions on the wards."

"Praise God," Reverend Beals exclaimed. "Christian nationals are taking over. God's work will go on even after we're gone."

The group around the table finished their meeting and ended in a time of prayer and praise to God.

In due time, Jean packed up her belongings and set out in the jeep with Kissen to her newly appointed post. Her role required supervision of thirty staff and the well-being of the children, and overseeing the clinic attached to the school property. As well, she'd purchase school supplies, collect school fees from the parents, and balance the books. She also stepped into the Mission Treasurer's job, and this demanded sending quarterly reports to the head office in Kansas. Bill Pease spent time schooling Jean in her new role.

"I just hope I can do as good a job as you," she said, looking at Bill's neat entries in the ledger.

"You will," he said.

Lenora gave Jean a tour of the school, the dorms and the classrooms, where children eyed her with curiosity. Her managerial skills enabled her to settle in quickly to her new position.

After the first year, she penned the following letter to her church back home.

Nazarene Christian Coeducational School,
Chikhli, District of Buldana, Maharashtra, India. 1967–68

Dear Friends,

Greetings from India and especially from NCC School this hot season morning. The windows and doors are closed to preserve some of the fresh, cool air that came in during the night.

Though it is April, Christmas cards are still coming to remind me of the many friends God has given. Thank you for remembering me once again, and most of all for remembering me before the throne of God.

One day in the hospital, a non-Christian said to me, "We call and call on our gods and they do not answer, but every time you Christians call on your God, He hears and answers." Praise be to His worthy name. He does hear every prayer, and the results we shall see one day.

One year at the school is nearly finished now. It has been full to the brim, and what a change it is to have, instead of patients and nurses at the hospital, 175 boarding students and seventy-five day scholars on the compound each day. It has been a privilege to work with fifteen national workers here—the teachers, a matron for the girls' dorm, a housefather for the boys' dorm, a maintenance man, a buyer for food and supplies (you should see our store rooms, full of wood, grain, chilies, etc.), and a nurse who takes care of the students and also patients who come from the surrounding villages.

It is not enough to take care of the illnesses, feed the students three meals a day and have a well-organized school, but we pray that God will move among us until each child will not only give his or her heart to Jesus, but they will learn to walk the Highway of Holiness with the King of kings.

This year, it would have gladdened my heart to see much more, but I do praise God, for He has given some outstanding victories. We appreciate your prayers for each staff member and each student.

Most of all, it has been a blessed year because I knew I was in God's will. My heart has been full of His praises, for although the way is sometimes difficult, and the results not visible in the measure we wish to see, still we can press on. Looking unto Jesus, for one of these days we shall not see in part, but the whole.

May God bless you, each one, and may we say, *"Revive us again that thy people may rejoice in Thee"* (Psalm 85:6).

Sincerely in His service,

Jean Darling

The next day, Jean stood with Kissen and Amrut watching workmen tackle the final phase of the preparation for two wells. The drills hummed as the men held them steady. A shout of joy went up when water gushed forth. Kissen danced a little jig on the spot.

"No more water shortage. This is very good, Sister, yes?"

"It is, Kissen. God is taking care of us. Now the water pumps can be installed and we're all set."

Ankita, a widow, and Jabbu, her daughter—both of whom assisted Jean with housekeeping, cooking and cleaning—came toward them with big smiles. "God is good," Ankita exclaimed.

Jean watched Ankita and rejoiced for her. She and her daughter had been saved for ten years, and Jean marveled at the evidence of the Holy Spirit in their lives.

"We will go and finish the cooking," Ankita said. "Come, Jabbu."

"That's good. I'll see you later. I'm going to the school." Jean looked over to the fence that surrounded the bungalow. Her dog Roxie sat, ears upright waiting for her command.

"Roxie, come, come." The Alsatian dog bounded across the quadrangle. "I'm so glad to have you," Jean said, as she petted the dog. "You're a great companion. Do you know that?" Roxie wagged her tail as if she did.

The dog had belonged to Doctor Cox, and he had given it to Hilda Moen. But now she belonged to Jean. "My constant companion and guard dog, aren't you?" Jean said.

She told the dog to stay at the gate, and Roxie obediently sat with her ears perked up, watching Jean walk across the school compound.

"Hello, boys." Jean stopped to speak to a group chatting to each other in the play area.

"Where's Roxie, Auntie?"

"You know where she is, don't you. She's just inside the gate waiting for me. You see how obedient she is. That's the way God wants us to be to Him." The boys listened to Jean.

"Why is she always obedient?" Jay asked.

"She pays attention when I talk to her."

"And that's how we have to be," Kirin said, his big brown eyes fixed on Jean.

"Very good, Kirin."

Jean moved on and entered the school building. She met the housefather coming down from the dorms with his two-year-old son. They exchanged pleasantries and she continued on her way, checking in classrooms, speaking with teachers, and then going upstairs to the dormitories. All was well. Coming out into the playground, she smiled as she heard children mimicking her commands to Roxie. *Their English accents are so cute,* she thought.

A routine had been established at the school, and Jean along with her staff found it a rich experience to visit some of the village churches on Sundays, and some of the non-Christian scholar's homes during the week.

"Hello Auntie," "Good morning, Auntie," several children called out to Jean as she entered the Sunday school classroom in the village church. The teacher greeted Jean and then addressed the children.

"Do you remember what we talked about last week?" she asked. The children, eager to respond, waved their hands in the air. "Yes, Janu, you tell us."

"We talked about praying and believing and I prayed for a baby brother, because I have five sisters, and God gave me a baby brother."

"That's wonderful news, Janu. Would you like to pray now and thank God?"

The little girl bowed her head and closed her eyes. "Dear Jesus, I asked you to give me a brother and you did. Thank you for this."

Although many of the parents were not Christian, they allowed their children to attend church, and the Christians silently thanked God for the opportunity to share the good news. Children learned to quote scripture, to sing and to pray.

They are so natural, and pray from their hearts, Jean observed as they interacted with their teacher.

Monday afternoon, Jean and Jabbu prepared to make cookies and candies for Independence Day celebrations. "We should make at least five hundred and fifty cookies," Jean told Jabbu. "Then we'll have enough for prayer day, too."

"Yes, there will be many visitors," Jabbu said, as she opened the fridge door and peered in. "Oh, no. We have no eggs."

"Not to worry," Jean announced cheerfully. "Powdered eggs and cake mixes will work just as well."

In the bungalow kitchen, the two pulled bowls, wooden spoons and other cooking utensils out of the cupboards and set to work. The end result produced the five hundred and fifty cookies and three hundred pieces of white fudge flavoured with cinnamon.

Independence Day celebrations took place on August 15. The children were excited to be excused from regular classes and instead paraded in their best clothes in the quadrangle and sang songs. Jabbu, Ankita, Kissen and Amrut helped Jean serve the special tea to the visitors, children, and teachers.

Always resourceful, and with certain foods hard to come by, Jean wrote in one of her letters:

If you find some instant packages that do not have to be cooked for a long time, I wish you would include them in a parcel. Nothing like imposing, is there. Sweets of all kinds are $1.00 per kilo (2.2 lbs), and that is very expensive for here...

Writing on, she shared the challenges regarding the electricity supply:

The electricians have been here wiring for phase-three electricity—we've had only one phase in some of our bungalows. The mechanic is overhauling our Jeep station wagon and the typewriter maintenance man is checking and repairing all the typewriters.

Tomorrow, I will start working and cleaning for Wednesday. All the missionaries will come...about sixteen or seventeen.

Carolyn had a man bring some wild pig, so we'll roast it on Tuesday, then heat the rest up on Wednesday…

Such were the responsibilities and diversities of her job—the equivalent of a housewife many times over. Jean finished writing, and for a moment gazed out of the window. Roxie, who had been lying at her feet, looked up, her head cocked to one side and her bright eyes inquisitive.

"Yes Roxie, I'm missing Jabbu. She had to go back to Basim. Let's hope our new girl will settle in."

Jean sighed and reached for the ledgers. Feeling tired and drained, she bent over her desk, scrutinizing the records. Everything had to balance out for the auditors who were arriving the next day, and she had to complete the treasures report by the end of the week.

She stopped and bowed her head. "Dear Lord, I wonder how I will manage, but on the other hand it's good to know the date I need to get this done. Today my mind is so tired, and I cannot think as I should. Please help me." The prayer uttered, she set to with renewed strength. Speaking every morning in the chapel services over the past week had been invigorating, but at the same time she surmised her tiredness stemmed from that.

The books finished, Jean stood and stretched, then made her way to the kitchen. Roxie trotted behind her and lay down at the kitchen door. She knew she was allowed no further. "Hello, Sister." Rita stood at the stove stirring a pot of curry.

"It smells delicious, Rita," Jean said.

"I know you like curry. The rice is in this pot," she said, pointing to a smaller saucepan on the stove.

Jean thanked Rita and complemented her on her good work. "You remember I have to go to Akola in the morning," she reminded her.

The girl nodded. "I remember I take care of everything." Rita turned the gas off under the pots. "I will go home now, and be here early in the morning."

Kissen drove Jean to Akola early the next day. She had been asked to give a presentation to a group of health care professionals on the methods she had used to start the nursing school in the Reynolds Memorial Hospital in Basim. News of its success had roused much interest. She did this gladly, giving useful information to the team, who were looking for direction in implementing a nursing school in their own hospital.

"Well that was an interesting day," said Doctor Evelyn Whittoff as she sat in the back of the Jeep. Doctor Whittoff had been working in Akola for a few weeks and had also presented at the conference.

Jean murmured an agreement. She fought to stay alert as Kissen drove, but eventually her head fell forward and she slept. She awoke as Kissen pulled into the school complex.

Roxie came bounding to the Jeep and greeted Jean with little yelps and vigorous tail-wagging, in between jumping up to lick her face. Jean laughed. "Did you miss me, my friend?" she said as she ruffled the dog's fur.

Thanking Kissen, Jean and Evelyn went into the bungalow, where they had supper and relaxed before going to bed.

A beam of bright sunlight pierced its way in between the curtains in Jean's bedroom. She rolled over and looked at her clock. Time to get up. Lenora and Bill Pease were back from furlough and ensconced in the guest bungalow for a few days, before heading out to man the new work in Auragabad.

Washed and dressed, she hurried out to the kitchen.

"Good morning," Evelyn greeted her.

"To you, too," Jean said. "Yes Roxie, I know you want out." Roxie stood wagging her tail and gave an excited bark as Jean let her out into the enclosure to the rear of the bungalow. "Doctor Cox and his wife arrive today for a visit. All is excitement and work," she added with a grin.

"Yes. I wonder if I should ride back to Basim with them."

"I'd love you to stay for the week as planned," Jean said, as she picked up the cup of tea Evelyn had poured.

"As planned, it shall be."

"Would you like to join me for devotions after breakfast?" Jean asked. Her companion smiled and nodded. Breakfast finished, the two women took their dishes to the sink. Rita came in at that moment and insisted on washing them.

"You have plenty to do, Sister," she announced with a cheerful smile.

Jean thanked Rita, and the two friends retreated to the living room. They checked the daily devotional reading for the day and opened their bibles. Jean paused for a moment.

"Jabbu is begging me to take her back," she told Evelyn. "But Rita is doing well; she can iron, do laundry and wash dishes, but is not the help Jabbu was. I taught Jabbu so much, and I miss her. However, it is all in the hands of the Lord, and I just pray for his direction to lead me into which way I should go."

"Let's pray about the situation now," Evelyn said. "It would be hard for Rita if you dismissed her, wouldn't it?"

"For sure. Why don't we pray for both of them and ask God to meet their needs?"

At the end of their prayer time, Jean took Evelyn on a tour of the classrooms and the dorms. She introduced her to members of staff, and during her stay they often popped over to the bungalow for an evening visit. The clinic located on the school grounds, and manned by a missionary doctor and nurse, was open to the villagers and the school children alike, and there Evelyn saw the staff in action tending to a variety of ailments.

Another Christmas approached. It was December, 1969, and Jean thrilled at the excitement of the children as preparations took place in the school. There were choir practices, nativity plays and special readings to be practiced. Parents came to see their children perform, and staff prayed the gospel message would penetrate hearts.

Jean wrote a hurried note to her mother:

December 6, 1969
Dear Mom,
The days are slipping by so fast, and it will be Christmas before we know it. I have enjoyed the letters from you all. Thank you. Wish I could write to everyone separately, but it is

not possible again this year. You have a wonderful Christmas. I enjoyed your letter telling me of your new apartment and the possibility of getting one on the first floor.

Tomorrow I will decorate my dining room before prayer day on Wednesday…there will be twenty-two of us.

Our vacation time is from the 23rd to January 5. During that time, I will go to Bombay to the wedding of Doctor Bhujbal, who has been working to relieve Doctor Witthoff. She is a lovely young lady, as well as a good doctor, and we hate to lose her, but she is marrying a doctor, so there is the possibility that the two of them may come to Basim to serve.

The single ladies will have Christmas together at Mrs. Myatt's. She is a widow. Her husband drowned while they were on their honeymoon…

Merry Christmas to you all,

Love, Jean

"Oh, dear. I will have to improvise." Jean stared at the lights in the bungalow. They stayed on for a few seconds and then went off for ten minutes or more. She needed to get ready for church, and the faulty electricity supply meant no hot water for showering. She quickly filled a couple of pots with water and put them on the gas burner—a sponge-down would have to do. While the water heated, she stepped outside with Roxie. The dog chased around the enclosure and Jean sat on the wooden seat on the back porch and gazed at the sunrise.

"What an amazing God you are," she whispered, as she watched the sky aglow with deep red hues that slowly faded to a pale yellow. *Such breath-taking patterns.* Her thoughts turned to her loving family back home in Canada. *I must write soon to thank them for their generous Christmas parcels.* And so she did.

December 16, 1969

Dear Mom & all,

Waiting for the Peases to come for breakfast…

This week, three parcels from Ralph, your parcel Audrey,

and four yesterday from Grace and Mom. What a supply. Ralph
sent cheese and hams, and oh how wonderful it is to have these
for Christmas. Audrey, that was just what I needed. Thank you,
thank you all…

A few days before Christmas, Jean wrote her final letter of the year,
telling her family the many activities going on at the school, of the gifts
that the school children had received, of her attendance at the children's
Christmas concert, and her outreach to the district and how she had
invited the Superintendent of Police, a Hindu, and his family, for an
evening meal, then the organization of a Christmas tea for the staff. She
also told of her sermon preached in a church some twelve miles from
the school.

With the letter completed, Jean travelled to Basim. There she had
treasurer's work to do in the hospital office and to make deposits at the
bank. She returned to the school, seventy miles away, to have Christmas
dinner with the school children who were unable to go home for
Christmas. So ended her work for 1969.

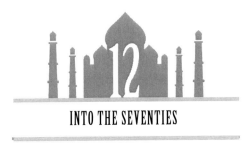

INTO THE SEVENTIES

"GOOD MORNING." PRESCOTT BEALS, THE DISTRICT Superintendent, greeted Jean with his usual smile as he stepped into the school office. He had been staying in one of the bungalows on the school grounds, overseeing a series of special meetings for the children with missionaries from the Alliance Church.

"Good morning to you, too," Jean said. "The Lewellens have already left. They wanted an early start."

"The meetings were excellent and the children loved Pastor Lewellen's illustrations. What a clever way to tell the gospel stories."

"Yes, using his gifts," Jean said. "Shall we go?"

Together, they walked over to the classrooms. Entering the grade two boys' class, they were treated to a recitation of the times table, with each child trying to outdo the other.

"Well done, boys," Reverend Beals exclaimed.

Before he could say more, Kirin shot his hand up.

"Yes, Kirin," his teacher said.

"Auntie, are you coming to have supper with us tonight?" he asked, looking at Jean.

Sometime ago, Jean had made that promise, and that night she kept it.

Organizing the children according to age for a day away at camp was next on the agenda. The children aged fifteen and over would go on day one, and the younger ones the next day.

Lined up in the compound, excited teenagers waited to board the rented bus, with Amrut at the wheel. Other children were taken by their parents. On day two, the same procedure occurred with the younger children.

In February, the missionaries and some of the nationals went for their own time of camping. Geraldine came, and Jean was happy to have time with her friend. They enjoyed some great meetings, but were not too thrilled with the nonexistent toilet facilities.

"This is not my idea of fun," Geraldine wailed as she made her way to the backside of the tent.

"Well, at least the holes are dug, and we do have a little grass matting around them for privacy," Jean teased.

Camping over, the missionaries, twenty in all, went to Buldana and congregated there for district assembly, followed by prayer day. The Peases were now ready to head up a new work in Auragabad, and Jean had been asked to continue her administrator's role at the school.

The group tucked in to the luncheon served in the bungalow.

"Jean, your mother's Christmas cake is delicious," Lenora said, as she helped herself to another piece.

"Yes, and thank goodness it always arrives on time and keeps well for weeks."

"Hello there." Reverend Beals approached the two women with a smile. He spoke to Jean. "We'll have to leave early tomorrow. How about nine?"

"That's fine. I'll let Amrut know."

The sun was high in the sky when they drove out the next morning. Amrut knew the route well to Auragabad, some ninety miles away.

Reverend Beals sat in the passenger seat and Bill Pease, Jean and the Indian District Superintendent sat in the back. The Nazarenes had purchased land in Auragabad, and this would be the location for Bill and Lenora Pease to start a new work. The goal—to build a church, a parsonage, and possibly a reading room. Jean accompanied the group in order to handle any money transactions.

Upon her return, Jean checked her mail, anxious to know whether her request for some time off had been acknowledged by head office in Kansas, and yes, it had. She immediately mailed a letter to her family, letting them know of the tentative plans.

> February 28, 1970
> …February has slipped by unnoticed. Oh, how fast the days fly. Your letters came and I was so glad to hear from you again…
>
> I had written to Doctor Phillips at Kansas City about my furlough and, since all is so uncertain, offered to go for three months during this winter, or wait until the spring of '71 for a regular furlough. He says he approves of either one. If the council members here are in agreement, I will plan to come in November through to January and then come back. That would give me rest enough during the hot season. I would not do deputation work at home, but would have to go to the Board meeting in January. I think this is wise for all concerned, but will wait for the council to decide on our prayer day, March 13…Anyway, all is out of our hands and I wait for leading…

With approval from head office, council met and decided on dates. Doctor Speicher and Jean could take three months' leave, and Carolyn Myatt a year.

Jean informed her family that at the end of October or early November, she'd arrive home:

> …I think Carolyn is leaving at the same time so we can travel together. We'll get a round-world ticket, so will no doubt

go by Singapore, Hong Kong and Japan… The near east is still dangerous, so we'll not go near there…

Must run now. Have had many interruptions…

"The fridge is fixed, Sister." Amrut stood in the doorway.

Jean looked up. "The fridge challenges us, even though we've upgraded to a better electrical system," she said. "Thank you, Amrut, for taking care of it again."

"Now I will help Kissen fix Miss Geraldine's car," Amrut said. "He already has the engine out. I hope we get it back in." He grinned.

Jean laughed. "You will," she said. "Geraldine only has two more days before she goes back to Basim." Finishing the work at her desk, she went to the kitchen, where Rita, the new help, sprinkled liberal doses of powder on the kitchen shelves.

"How are you getting on, Rita?"

"I'm nearly done. I do hope it will get rid of them."

"You're doing a good job," Jean encouraged, "and by tomorrow, no more cockroaches, right? Did Ravi come back from the market?"

"Not yet."

"Tell him all the produce will have to go in the school kitchen for the night."

"Yes, Sister. I will take care and sweep up the cockroaches."

Two days later, Geraldine returned to the Reynolds Memorial Hospital, and the following week Jean set out for Basim in her little car. Committee and treasurer's work demanded her attention. But soon they'd all be heading to the hills.

Driving back, her thoughts turned to repairs that needed to be done at the school. In her mind she planned a to-do list, and knew Kissen and Amrut would faithfully tackle the work. Then, the joint committee would meet tomorrow with the Indian Advisory Board and the Executive Committee of Missionaries. They'd be focusing on the annual task of relocating the pastors. But more important at that moment was the message she would deliver in church on Easter Sunday morning, and so she contemplated on that.

The busy days went by, and in April the school year drew to a close. The buildings, emptied of their boisterous occupants, stood silent in the scorching sun. Jean wrote to her home church telling of the exodus.

April 15, 1970
Dear Friends,

From early morning, excitement has run high with boys and girls making a grand exodus from the boarding school. Fathers and brothers carry tin trunks and rolls of bedding. Today, school is out for summer vacation.

At noon, a boy, followed by his brother, came to my office weeping as if his heart would break. His father had not come, nor sent money for their bus fare home. I tried to console him and said, "It's okay. You are a big boy and you and your brother can work in my garden today and then you will have your fare to go home." He smiled and without hesitation he took the shovel and basket and went to work.

After a while, my doorbell rang. The boys greeted me with the words, "Our father has come." These words spoke to my heart and I praised God that my father had come.

With the end of the school year, I find my thoughts and yearly greetings speeding their way over the mountains, across the land and sea to my friends who have been so faithful to me one more year. Thank you for remembering me with letters, greetings, gifts and prayers. I know it costs to remember, and words cannot express my appreciation. Surely we are workers together with Him.

This year, again, activities have filled the days to overflowing, with study, games, programs and the routine of daily living. The girls and the boys often played pranks, fought and made up. A few days ago, a group of boys ran away to the nearby well to swim, and others to partake of the neighbor's mangoes. I couldn't allow them to think they were just normal boys, up to typical mischief. After I explained the error of their ways, they willingly worked to pay for the already digested mangoes and surprised the farmer by asking forgiveness and giving him the money, which he accepted reluctantly.

However, the spiritual results cause us to fall on our faces, and to praise God for the outpouring of His Spirit upon us this year in Chikhli. In October, the Spirit came upon Pastor Bansod with a new challenge and burden for revival. November was a month of special meetings for the Marathi area. People were open and walked in the Light. Three teenage girls, daughters of staff, obeyed and prayed and revival came. In January, Reverend Beals, who spent many years in India as a missionary, held meetings for the church and school. Many responded to his message of love, and met God with definite victory. It was a miracle before our eyes to see one after another admit their need and pray through. The Spirit still prevails and the church is reaching out to the villagers…We realize this is only the beginning, and Satan does not sleep, so we must continue to fight the good fight of faith. We appreciate your prayers, especially for the young people as they carry the burden along with the adults…

Kissen and Amrut sat in the bungalow, each drinking a glass of lemonade. The steady whirl of the fans hanging from the ceiling seemed desperately trying to combat the 120-degree temperature. Jean sat opposite them, studying her to-do list. She could feel the perspiration trickling down her back. She drank more lemonade and then spoke.

"A great deal of repair work is needed. I know you two will oversee the work and get as much done as you can before you break for the summer. The wooden fence around the back of the school has to be replaced with metal posts."

"We will do that," Kissen said, "and we will string wire between them."

"It will stop the villagers leaving their goats to eat our grass, too," Amrut added.

Jean studied the list. "A new engine house for the pump has to be built. The materials have been ordered for that and for the girls' bathrooms. The three toilets arrived yesterday, as you know. What about the school refrigerator? Did the repair team from Hyderabad City pick it up?"

"Yes," Amrut said. "We helped load it into their truck."

Kissen and Amrut, with cheerful determination, led a team of workmen in tackling the repairs and upgrades. By early May, most of the tasks were completed.

In sweltering heat, Jean drove to Basim; she had book work to do at the hospital, and from there she wrote to her mother:

> May 12, 1970, Basim
> Dear Mom,
> Have been at the hospital since yesterday and today am working, but am almost finished—will leave this evening and fly away to the hills. I am really weary—the heat is unbearable—everyone looks washed out…
> Sunday was Mother's Day. We had a beautiful service in Chikhli church. They asked me to pray the closing prayer, and I prayed for you as well as all the mothers represented and present. People always comment on how hospitable I am, so I tell them it was my mother who taught me…so you get the credit for that. I appreciate your example as a mother. Trust you keep well and we can have a nice visit when I come home.

By the third week in May, thirty missionaries were housed in bungalows and boarding houses in the mountains. The higher altitude gave the group relief from the sweltering heat. Jean stood on the verandah with Geraldine, gazing into the valley below. They both exclaimed wonder at the same moment. Before them, a magnificent rainbow arched between two majestic mountain peaks.

"God's creation," Jean said softly.

"Indeed."

They stayed there, breathing in the cool air. Feeling refreshed in body and spirit.

Although the missionaries had escaped the heat, they attended conferences that zeroed in on their areas of ministry. They gave reports of the progress God had allowed, and shared ideas.

Jean, along with other medical missionaries, listened intently as one of the doctors presented progress in the Satara district. A knock on the door interrupted his discourse. The hostess of the boarding facility entered the room and apologized for the interruption.

"We've received an urgent request from the nearby hospital for type O blood," she announced. "There's a little Tibetan boy hemorrhaging after his surgery. Is there anyone who could donate?" She glanced around the room.

Without hesitation, Geraldine, Hilda, and Jean volunteered. With Geraldine at the wheel of the Jeep, they drove to the hospital and gave a pint each.

Once a week, while on respite from the plains, missionaries from different organizations reached out to the little community to spread the good news of the gospel. On Wednesday of that same week, a number of Nazarene missionaries stood behind a long table filled with sandwiches, little cakes, and cookies. They had traversed a winding path up the side of the mountain and entered the community centre of a small village.

Two women dressed in colourful saris stood hesitantly at the door.

"Come in," Jean greeted them with a warm smile. They moved forward slowly, and glanced around the room. Jean invited them to sit at one of the tables.

"We're expecting a lot of people," she said. "Here they come." She clapped her hands as a group of ten to twelve people came in. Soon the room was crowded. Geraldine and Hilda mingled with the folks and engaged them in conversation. Brother Beals stood at the front and with his charming personality officially welcomed everyone.

The villagers visibly relaxed as they listened to a gospel trio and watched humorous little skits. By the time the missionaries served tea, God's love had affected everyone in the room.

The respite over, many of the missionaries travelled to Bombay to attend to personal necessities, such as dental checkups and the purchase of supplies. As Jean exited a store with Geraldine, she said, "I'm so anxious to get back to work and see the children again."

"And Roxie," Geraldine added.

"Oh, yes. Dear Roxie, she practically eats me alive when I return. But Kissen is so good. He looks after her well." She stopped and looked at her friend. "Imagine, only sixteen to seventeen more weeks and I'll be in Canada. How good it will be to see my family again. It's funny, in a way—we want to go home, but we long to come back."

An excited company of children laughed and chatted and called out to each other as they lined up at the registration tables with their parents. The silent school buildings once again resounded with life.

"Hello, Jay, Kirin. How are you?" Jean walked along the lines, greeting the children.

"Auntie, my baby brother is walking now." Excitedly, the children clamoured to tell Jean their family news. A surge of joy engulfed her as she looked at the animated faces around her.

"Where's Roxie, Auntie?"

Jean recalled Roxie's enthusiastic greeting at seeing her again. She had decided to leave her in the bungalow until the children settled down. "She'll visit you tomorrow," she assured them.

"Good morning, Sister," the housemaster said to Jean. "So much excitement."

Jean laughed. "I agree." She indicated she needed to speak to him privately, and they both stepped to the side.

"I have to go to Basim to take care of the books. I'll be back tomorrow."

"That is fine. The housemother is here for the girls, and all the teachers have arrived."

Jean made her away across the compound and back to her bungalow. Uppermost in her mind was the shortage of food. Kissen had kept a good supply of grain in the store room, but other foods were hard to come by. The loss of crops and produce due to a lack of rain was quite significant. She had the job of applying for permits in order to get rations for the children. "We have two hundred and fifty hungry mouths to feed," she announced to Roxie as she entered the bungalow.

Driving out of the grounds, she marveled at the work Kissen and Amrut had achieved during her time away. In spite of the heat, they had managed, with the help of the gardener and groundsmen, to plant flowers and dig holes for a row of trees. The new fence was in place, and the goats had been kept out. A green lawn had started to take shape. Rain had fallen mid-June, resulting in the flowers blooming in the school gardens. The motor for the main pump that served the bungalows still awaited repair, but the gardener assured Jean he would fill her bucket each day from the small pump in the back garden. The pumps supplying the school were in working order, but still, she reckoned they'd have to be prudent.

School life resumed, and through careful administration and some improvising with recipes, they were able to provide the children three good meals a day.

Some disconcerting news about her mother's health had Jean willing the weeks away. Sitting at her desk, she responded to the family letter.

July 29, 1970
Dear Mom and all,
This is Wednesday…I received your letters. I trust you are feeling better, Mom. You must have a lot of pain. Is it a form of arthritis in your hip and back? Yes, I do pray that God will give you relief.
…Your time seems interesting, Audrey. I thought, how like the Lord to supply you with a car…the days are sailing by, and three months from now I will be on my way home…

Her concerns remained with more news of her mother's troubles.

August 3, 1970
Mom, I hope your back is better and that you are feeling well. Did the doctor tell you why your feet are swelling?
Doctor Speicher came through yesterday while I was in church. She went on to Buldana on some business, but will drop in on her way home. We had prayer day in Buldana last

week. The cars gave us trouble, but otherwise it was a lovely day. Next prayer day is the 26th. Doctor Speicher's sister is coming just for a year. She is a lovely person. She and her husband were missionaries in Alaska for years…

The letter finished, Jean turned her thoughts to her work. It was time to go.

The teachers sat around the table in the small conference room for their weekly meeting. Jean listened to a young teacher who, with a worried frown, expressed concerns about the number of children in the school.

Jean acknowledged her concerns with a nod. "It is true our numbers have increased, and keeping tabs on them all is a challenge. As well as their education, we have to address their overall health, see that they bathe regularly, change their clothes, and above all else that none gets head lice. I did find lice in two of the boys yesterday. But the necessary measures were taken. Most of all, we should not worry, but realize God has given us a work to do."

The housemaster spoke. "How important that is. I think, too, that we should take note of any child scratching his or her head and examine it at once. Do let Sister or myself know immediately."

"And bedbugs, too, can be a huge problem. I took one back to the bungalow after sitting in a chair in the boys' dorm," Jean said. "We must always spray so that none of this gets out of control."

Other issues were discussed, decisions made, and the meeting adjourned after they prayed.

On Friday evening, Jean travelled to Auragabad. She had been asked by the newly appointed pastor to preach in his fledgling church. Services were held in his home. She thrilled as she met with the pastor and saw the beginnings of the new ministry the Nazarenes had prayed for. She recalled the day they had visited to seal the purchase of the property. The Peases were now settled in a small bungalow, spearheading this new work in between trips to Buldana and Chikhli on mission business. They welcomed Jean into their little home, where she would sleep for the two nights.

Over the next two days, she preached in four services, delivering a message of encouragement. As well, the Peases drove her and the pastor to homes in different parts of the city, where she met joyful believers.

On the Sunday evening, the Peases invited the pastor and his wife to join them for an evening meal. They sat around the table discussing the services, and agreeing that God had been present in all of them.

Jean spoke to the pastor. "There are wonderful prospects here, and we will continue to pray that God will guide you, and that His Spirit will work among the people."

"Ah, yes," the young pastor said. "We are so happy with the evidence of God in our midst already." He looked fondly at his wife and she nodded in agreement.

Jean smiled. "Next week is the preachers' meeting and exams. Our housefather and new manager will be attending. So I will have my hands full overseeing the boys."

"But you'll manage," Lenora said with a smile.

The meal finished, the pastors left, and Jean went to bed soon after. She needed to get an early start back to the school in the morning.

The rains fell as she drove back. This turned her thinking to the snakes that would be surfacing in the garden. She breathed a silent thank you for Kissen, who checked the garden and bungalows with diligence. He had deftly removed a baby cobra from her dining room the week before.

On August 18, 1970, Jean penned her usual letter to her mother and family. In the relative comfort of the bungalow, she settled down and wrote:

> Thank you for your letter, Mom, and the lovely parcel of milk, mixes, candy, cheese and coffee, etc. Everything arrived intact. Thank you so much…

Her letter told of the missionary outreach to surrounding villages, and how a capable driver had driven her and Carolyn through heavy rain in order for Jean to speak in a village some forty miles away from the school.

On August 30, Jean's sister, Grace, read the letter in its entirety to their mother, and on that same day, their mother passed away.

September 6, Jean again mailed a letter to the family, not knowing yet of her mother's passing. In it, she wrote:

>...The days are flying fast. Seven weeks from yesterday, I will be leaving Chikhli and will stay in Akola for a couple of days for permits, etc. I arrive in the USA most likely on November 1.
>...I trust you are feeling better, Mom. The weather should be beautiful now.
>Love & prayers, *Jean*

My little car knows its way to Basim without my help, Jean thought as she drove along. She arrived midday and went straight to the Business Manager's office.

Ely greeted her with a big smile. "The books are ready, Sister. I tallied all the figures and I pray I got it right."

"I'm sure you did. You have been a very good student," Jean said. *And,* she thought, *so teachable and respectful.* "Why don't you take a break, Ely, and I'll check the annual financial statement. I should be done in an hour or so." Jean set to work, and everything balanced. She complimented Ely on his work and returned to Chikhli in the pouring rain.

The rain eased off mid-week, and Rita helped Jean with washing sheets from the guestrooms. As they went out to hang them on the line, another downpour started.

"Well, we'll have to hang them up inside," Jean said. Together they strung lines in the guestroom, the living room, and bathroom, and then turned on the ceiling fans.

That done, Jean, with her umbrella, walked over to the guest bungalow, where Geraldine Chappell had started cleaning.

"The back bedroom's done," Geraldine called out.

"Great. I'll start in the dining area, if you want to work on the other bedroom," Jean said.

They were preparing the bungalow for the Greers, who were returning after furlough.

"Did you know they are driving from Jerusalem, through Iran and Pakistan, and then into North India?" Jean asked.

"Yes, that is quite the jaunt, especially this time of year, with the rains so heavy."

"Quite so. When I left Basim, there were 1,500 people in that area alone washed out of their homes. Many of them slept in the church. The hospital and the Famine Relief fund handed out grain and other supplies. I don't think there were any Christians among the people who came for help. Praise God for the opportunity once again to witness."

"Amen."

A few hours later, the bungalow now clean, the women returned to Jean's living room for refreshments. "I'll head back to Basim in the morning," Geraldine announced. "Do you know we're short-staffed at the hospital?"

"Yes, I know." Jean gave a wry grin. "I heard they may assign me back there on my return. I'd hate to leave here in the middle of a turnover, but," she announced with a sigh, "I shall go wherever they send me. I will suggest the move not be done until school is out and the hot season has arrived. On the other hand, I cannot dictate, but must wait on God to work out His plan and make it plain."

The September 6th letter crossed over the sea to Canada, and as it did the letter from Canada winged its way to India, arriving on Monday, September 7, informing Jean of her mother's passing.

Jean replied immediately.

September 8, 1970

Dear Grace & Audrey,

Your letter of September 1 arrived today. I have not received the one from the day before, so do not know the details of what happened. The Peases had come and gone. After they left, I opened my mail and was thankful to read it by myself. I am anxious to know what happened. I understand she went to the hospital on Friday, August 21. I was worried when she wrote before and said she had fluid in her lungs… Anyway, she has gone to be with Jesus, and that is the most important thing. To think I just wrote last evening that I only had seven weeks left.

I will still come home and stay part-time with Audrey and part-time with you, Grace.

It is well that she did not suffer too much, but I am wondering what she did suffer with?

Anyway, she has gone first, and then we will go afterwards to meet her. What hope there is in God. With sorrow there is comfort from Him, and for that I praise Him. I wonder what letter she received from me. Was it the one where I mentioned taking care of her and reminded her of the time I took care of her in the hospital? What took her life? Did they tell you?

Well, Grace, you looked after her so well. Otto did too, and I am so grateful for that. It was so nice, Audrey, that you were home from Winnipeg this summer. You will all have these memories for the rest of your lives.

You will have an adjustment this year, Audrey, with your roommate Pauline now moved out and married. It will be a wonderful year for you with God, who will do more than you can imagine. You give up anything for Him and he will repay you in a thousand ways. Do not worry about finances or anything. God will supply your every need. He has given me so much more than I deserve, and He will continue to meet all our needs…

Well, I will write again when I hear more news… May God bless you always. I will see you soon. I will enjoy my time home with you, even though it will be different.

Love and prayers,

Jean

Dusk fell, and Jean sat in her living room. Thoughts of her mother occupied her mind. She wanted more than anything to go home at that moment, to be with her siblings—but she would not—she could not. She would stay at her post until October, when she was scheduled to leave.

A knock on the door interrupted her thoughts. Carolyn Myatt walked in. "Thought you might like some company," she said.

"Thank you so much. I appreciate it."

"I can stay the night, if you like."

Jean smiled. "Yes, I'd like that. You know, Carolyn, this has been a great opportunity to do some more witnessing. Some of our staff cannot understand why we do not wail and make a big noise when a loved one dies. A Buddhist lady dropped by this afternoon. Her daughter is a boarder here. I told her that Mom was ready to go to Jesus, and that if she believed in Him, she could have that same assurance. Nothing really matters, only that we are ready to meet Him."

"How true," Carolyn said.

The two had a quiet evening together. They talked, read the Bible, and had some prayer time. "I'll be getting up early," Carolyn said. "It's clinic day tomorrow, but I'll see you at lunchtime."

The next day was the missionaries' "get together" day. At the end of each month, all of those who were able gathered in the bungalow for lunch and fellowship.

Rita came from the kitchen and told Jean the lunch was ready. "I just have to make the tea, when they arrive."

"Thank you, Rita. They'll soon be here. I'll keep reading my cards until they come."

She picked up the next one on the pile. *So your sweet mother has gone,* Geraldine had written. A smile flittered across Jean's face as she read Doctor Speicher's note. *Don't you feel grateful for happy memories of her useful and good life, and what a fine mother she was to you and the brood?*

A knock on the door caused her to look up. "Come in," she called.

Doctor Whittoff poked her head around the door and said, "Hope we're not interrupting." She walked in, followed by Carolyn, the Peases and the Greers.

"Not at all. Lunch is ready. How was clinic?"

"The usual. But more importantly, how are you?" Doctor Whitthoff said.

"I'm fine, and I'm looking forward to going home, even though Mom won't be there. She's in a far better place."

Lenora gave her a hug, as did the others. The missionaries settled down to their customary lunch. Once a month, Carolyn and Doctor Evelyn Whitthoff were there to man the clinic. They shared that a number of the villagers had attended with a variety of ailments, and several of the children had been sent by the house-parents with minor health issues, too.

"I can hardly believe it. Six weeks from today, I fly to London and then on home to Canada," Jean said, as she handed a plate of her baked cookies to Carolyn.

"No more of your clever homemade recipes for a while," Lenora Pease noted. "But we pray God's peace for you and your family."

Jean nodded. "Thank you."

"How is the staff reacting to your news?" Paula asked.

"Those who know the Lord understand. Of course, they are sad for me and have promised to pray. But those who don't know Him are having a hard time. I find I'm consoling them. They can't understand how I can put aside my sorrow to do the work and take care of them and their needs. They can't understand why I'm not weeping and wailing. I tell them I'm sad and I will grieve, but because of my faith I'm assured that Mom is in heaven."

"Blessed assurance," Evelyn said. "Let's pray that many more will come to know Him through Jean's witness." The missionaries agreed, and after lunch prayed fervently for all those whom God had entrusted into their care.

In her next letter home, Jean shared with her siblings the reactions of the staff:

> They can see that we can spread sunshine in the midst of our sorrow. But we do not impose it on others. This is what they learned when Jack eventually died.
>
> I pray for you all that God will give you comfort. We do not have Mom anymore, but we have each other and we must carry on her work and witness, and be an example.
>
> With love,
> *Jean*

Much correspondence went back and forth in the days following. Jean wrote encouraging letters to her siblings:

> We have many wonderful memories of her, and she was an example to us. How fortunate we are to have had her for so long and to have had such a good mother. May we never forget the lessons she taught us by her example. On August 31, I read in my little devotional book, *Daily Strength for Daily Needs,* the following: "Now therefore keep thy sorrow to thyself and bear with good courage that which hath befallen thee." Then the poem:
>
> Go bury thy sorrow, the world has its share,
> Go bury it deeply, go hide it with care,
> Go bury thy sorrow let others be blessed,
> Go give them the sunshine and tell God the rest.
> Anon

Jean's thoughts were frequently with her family. She wrote words of comfort and assurance, telling them that as Christians they had opportunity to witness.

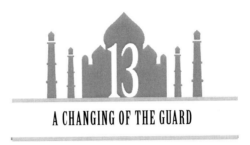

A CHANGING OF THE GUARD

I N FEBRUARY, 1971, AFTER A FEW MONTHS AT HOME, JEAN ONCE again returned to India. As the plane landed in Bombay, the old familiar feeling of coming home enveloped her. She knew Geraldine Chappell would be there to meet her, and as she came through the arrival lounge, she spotted Geraldine's tall figure among the crowd. The friends hugged and chatted nonstop as they travelled to Chikhli.

Back in the school compound, her dog Roxie went wild with excitement, almost knocking her over. "I'm back, Roxie," she laughed. "Yes, I'm back."

Entering the bungalow, Jean scanned the rooms, assessed the need, and within a day had her handyman and two boys whitewash the walls and paint the woodwork.

"You'll have it done in time," Geraldine assured her. The two were to go to Basim on the Friday and return to a houseful of guests—the

General Superintendent, Reverend Lawlor and his wife, the Peases, and the Greers.

"The Peases and the Greers are staying overnight," Jean said. "I'm going to put them in the other bungalow. They don't need to hear the rats that chew my roof half the night. They keep me awake, but I'd hate for guests to listen to that. I close both doors so the sound is lessened a bit."

Geraldine shuddered. "I don't know that I could be so matter-of-fact about it."

"Oh, well, that's India. Come on, let's have our dinner. I'm so blessed to have Tukaram. He cooks quite well, is learning to drive the car, and has a good deal of knowledge about electricity and the water pumps. Rita is doing well in the school, and of course Kissen and Amrut are treasures."

The daily routine prevailed again. In the middle of February, on a cool evening, Jean settled down to write to her sisters.

> February 15, 1971
> …Received your letters, Grace and Audrey, and I was glad to hear all the news. It seems like a dream that I was ever home, but how many wonderful memories I have…
>
> I had to expel four big boys from boarding last week. They continually disobeyed and thought we'd always let them get away with it. Their folk had to find somewhere for them to stay in the village. They can still come to school, but not board.
>
> Roxie is my constant companion. Right now, she is lying beside me as I write. The Lawlors were here yesterday to see the school, and had a noonday meal. I put Roxie in the bathroom. She was highly insulted, since I never, or very seldom, even tie her up, for she is most obedient.
>
> Today, camp meeting starts, so we are on the merry-go-round for one week. Tukaram will go to Buldana to help Doctor Whitthoff, who will have us for the two main meals, noon and night. We will have morning afternoon and tea at the Peases, for they live on the District centre property, where the camp will

be held. I will come and go, and sometimes have to stay at the school, so our nurse can get to some of the meetings. We have several boys with the mumps. They get up and run around. I hope they do not get colds, because the night temperatures are cold right now…

The busyness of school life never changed. Children sometimes got into mischief, and sometimes received reprimands from Jean and her staff. The pastor of the local church asked Jean to lead the young people and, ever willing, she prepared messages to share with them.

At six o'clock on a cool morning in mid-March, Jean sat on her verandah in her housecoat, playing her classical music on her tape recorder. The appearance of a car startled her. Roxie, who had been lying at her feet, stood and growled. She quickly grabbed her collar and went into the bungalow, where she pulled on her dress, ready to meet the unexpected visitor.

"Good morning, madam." A government official with three children came towards her.

"Good morning to you," Jean responded. "How can I help?"

"Madam, we are having a fair some fifteen miles from here. Would you have any tents we can borrow?"

Kissen, who had just come across the compound, offered to go to the school building with the government official. Tukaram offered too, and between them they piled three tents into the trunk. Jean gave the visitors orangeade and they went on their way.

"It's good that they felt comfortable to ask us. Let's pray they come to know Jesus." Jean spoke to Kissen. "Next week, I have to go to Basim. The nurses are writing their exams and I have to facilitate. It will be better if I leave early, before the temperature rises too much."

"Very busy for you," Tukaram observed, nodding his head as if in agreement to his own statement.

Jean smiled. "Yes, and before that we have our committee meeting here, regarding finances for the Indian District Assembly on Wednesday, and then the School Board meeting on Thursday. Ah well, Tukaram, it is all the Lord's business."

The following week, Jean stood at the front of the classroom in the Reynolds Memorial Hospital. A complement of twenty nurses sat at desks.

"Please, Sister Darling, could you explain exactly what they mean in paragraph two on the first page?" One of the student nurses asked the question as they read the instructions for their written exams.

"Let's go through this together. I will explain the rules to you. You may ask questions after I've finished. But once I give you the go-ahead to start, there must be no more talking."

The explanations completed, Jean took out her watch, laid it on the desk, raised her hand, and said, "Start." Only the scratching of pens and an occasional sigh were heard as the four-hour exam commenced.

Reflecting, Jean recalled back in 1946, when she had started the nursing school with four eager students. Now the school, recognized by the Nursing Board of India, required students to write the state exams. *God is faithful and His word is true,* she thought.

Changes were afoot. The Indian government had decreed that nationals should fill every management post throughout the Christian and foreign-built institutions. For the Christians, their goal had always been to step down once nationals were trained, and indeed, Nazarenes had already implemented some of the changes.

Jean glanced around the classroom at the rows of bent heads over the desks. Each student absorbed in the task at hand. Her thoughts flew to the school in Chikhli and another task that awaited her on her return. The government changes had come to the school, and that meant she had to clear out her desk and make room for the new manager, and for now she was to stay and assist him. A sensation of overwhelming gratitude swept over her as she realized the accomplishments achieved on the mission field, and all because of God's amazing grace.

The exams completed, she returned to Chikhli.

In her living room, she placed a tray with four glasses of lemonade on the coffee table. Bill and Lenora Pease were talking to their six-year-old son, Ricky. "You listen to Auntie Jean and do as she says," Bill reminded him.

The little boy nodded with his eyes fixed firmly on Roxie, who stood with tail wagging and head cocked to the side. The dog's bright eyes told the tale—she understood that here was a playmate for her.

"Can I play with Roxie now?"

Jean laughed. "Off you go, then." Dog and boy bounded into the backyard.

"We'll be back around noon on Friday. I hope the week won't be too tiresome for you," Lenora said.

"We'll be fine." The women hugged, and Jean walked to the gate with Lenora, while Bill waved to Ricky, who seemed not to notice as he threw Roxie's ball across the yard, yelling, "Fetch, fetch!"

The car pulled away, and Jean called out to Ricky. "Would you like to come over to the school and see the boys and girls?"

"Yes, please."

The two made their way across the compound, with Roxie in close proximity. Choruses of, "Hello Auntie," greeted them as they stepped into the school.

"Are you their Auntie, too?" Ricky asked.

"Yes, a sort of adopted aunt."

Ricky's attention was caught by three boys coming toward them, and Jean thought that possibly later he would be asking what "adopted" meant.

"Please, Auntie, you told us we have to forgive each other."

"Yes, Jay," Jean said.

"Well, Kiran has to ask your forgiveness. He called you an old deaf person, because you didn't answer last time when he said, 'Salam.'"

Jean hid the smile that threatened to rise. She looked at Kiran, who stood with head bowed, close to tears.

"Well, Kiran, I'm happy to forgive you if you want to ask for it," she said.

The little boy mumbled an apology. Jean bent down and gave him a hug. "All is forgiven. How about you show Ricky your classroom."

A big smile lit his face, and the boys set off with Jean and the other two close behind.

Back in the bungalow, Jean explained adoption to Ricky, pointing out how all who believed in Jesus had been adopted into God's family, and how as humans we sometimes adopt other human beings into our families.

The week ended, and Lenora and Bill came and took a reluctant Ricky back home. "I wish we could take Roxie," he said. And Roxie seemed to agree, giving little yelps as the family climbed into their Jeep and drove off.

April arrived, and with it the heat. Children prepared to go home for the summer break. Laughing, shouting, and teasing one another, they packed belongings and exited with their parents. The staff welcomed the peace. The heat sapped their strength. In the quiet of the bungalow, Jean penned a letter to her church family back home.

> Chikhli, District of Buldana, India
> April 17, 1971
> Dear Friends,
>
> It is time again to send yearly "hot season's greetings" across the sea to you, though many times during the year thoughts and prayers have taken their flight your way. Thank you, each one, for greetings, letters, parcels and other ways you have remembered me this year. I never cease to marvel at your faithfulness, interest and love. I realize we are "workers together" with Him. May God give us many souls to glorify His worthy name.
>
> The school year finished today. What silence after a year bulging with the activity of two hundred and thirty boarding students and sixty-five day scholars, most of whom are under fifteen years of age. May God go with each one to help them use in practical ways the truths they have learned. Some of them will not return, but most of them will be present when the merry-go-round starts for another school year.
>
> Since last July, Reverend S.P. Dongerdive, our treasurer for the India District, has been appointed by our Mission Council to be the manager of the school (I am now assistant manager). He not only loves the children and has talent communicating with them, but also is capable in administration and an example

to the staff. Surely God has given him to us, and we covet your prayers for him and all of us, as our nationals take more places of leadership.

While I was home on furlough in November, December and January, Mrs. Pease came from Buldana a couple of days a week and worked with him. For her contribution I am deeply grateful.

I missed seeing my mother by a few weeks, but it is wonderful that she did not have to suffer, for after three days of illness, she heard the celestial choir sing her welcome into the Eternal City. With the ache of sorrow was peace and comfort in Him, and sweet memories of her love and devotion.

Much was crammed into those three months, visiting loved ones, doing deputation work, especially in my home district of central Canada, plus my trip to Kansas City to meet with people in the Department of World Missions. Thank you, former and new friends, for the fellowship in Christ and for your many kindnesses to me while home. I returned back to India with a wealth of rich memories.

What a great privilege to have Doctor and Mrs. Lawlor visit us in India during the month of February. Doctor Lawlor held the India District Assembly and camp meetings. Victory came as our people recognized and responded to the word of God, which was given with unction. Mrs. Lawlor, dressed in an Indian sari, was also a special channel for the Holy Spirit as He sang, spoke, prayed, and loved through her. Surely it was a time of feasting for us all.

A young man named Anant Ingle was not completely truthful when he asked, and obtained, leave from the military to attend camp. He had two months' leave last year; during that time, he married. He lived at home with his father, a former Hindu priest, but now a preacher. He had attended services and became hungry, making a step forward during the meetings held last year by Reverend Beals. This time, he was afraid to leave before giving his life to Christ. He sobbed at the altar and confessed his sin. He left in victory with a heart dedicated to the Lord Jesus Christ. Please pray for him.

The weather stayed unusually cool up to mid-March, but then old "sol" poured its rays upon us until even the Indian people found it difficult to adjust to the sudden change. Even so, while trying to catch up with my work here, and helping out in the hospital at Washim (formerly Basim) in the business office with nurses' examinations, God has come with blessing, peace and poise as I try to do all as unto Him. What a joy to walk with Him.

As you pray for us, we pray also for you and our beloved church, that God will help us together accept in a greater measure the challenge to live the message of holiness, which alone will meet the need of the day.

May God bless each one of you.

Sincerely in His service,

Jean Darling

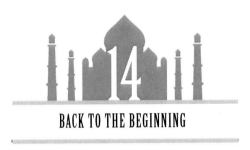

BACK TO THE BEGINNING

BY THE END OF APRIL, A THREE-DAY TREK BY TRAIN AND CAR HAD Jean, Geraldine, and many other missionaries stationed in the hills for rest, fellowship and prayer.

Toward the end of their stay, Jean and Geraldine walked along a mountain path. "I have a feeling I'll be back at the hospital for good before long," Jean said.

"Yes," Geraldine agreed. "They are short-staffed on several fronts."

"I've been asked to go to the hospital in July to teach the first- and second-year students. And also lead devotional time with all the nurses."

"It's amazing how God leads," Geraldine commented. "Did you ever think you'd do so much preaching when you first came? All those services in the Chikhli church, and then leading the young peoples' group."

Jean laughed. "No, but when God's in it, be prepared. I'm glad he gave me a head for math. The bookkeeping has been a challenge, but I do love working with figures."

Through the rest of the year, Jean travelled between the school and the hospital, attending to her allotted tasks. The September Council meeting held at the Reynolds Memorial Hospital engaged the members for several hours. Jean stifled a yawn as she listened to proposals regarding the roles of the group around the table. Doctor Speicher spoke. "We definitely need Jean back at the hospital," she said. "I propose she takes up administrative duties here as soon as can be arranged."

Back at the school, she once again penned a letter home.

Chikhli School
Thursday, September 23, 1971
…Well, our council meeting was longer than usual. There were so many items of business and so much discussion. I am transferred to the hospital again. This time, my assignment is to be hospital superintendent (administrator) and business manager. I will still be mission treasurer, so will have my hands full, but I do not need to face it yet. I will leave here at the end of October. There is much to do before then. Mrs. Pease will come here two days a week from Buldana. It is thrilling to see the Indian manager take over. He is such a godly man. I feel sad to leave all the children, but it does not seem real yet. These have been four and a half happy years.

Doctor Whittoff has gone to Ludhiana to have a specialist in neurosurgery check her. We trust it is nothing serious. She has been having dizzy spells. Lenora has gone with her.

I must have a bath and go to bed. I have to examine the patients in clinic tomorrow. Evelyn (Doctor Whittoff) was to be here. I will check all who come and refer any of whom I have doubts…

Friday, 10:00 am
Took five minutes off to finish this letter. It's a fairly big crowd in the clinic—have seen about twenty-five to thirty

patients so far. One child, three years—just skin and bones, like an old man, cannot even sit up. I suspect TB. It is terrible to see.

Must run,

Jean

"Only two more weeks, Roxie, and we are off to a new home." Jean bent down and stroked her dog's back.

Frantic banging on the door diverted her attention. "Sister, please come."

Jean hurried across the room and opened it. The gardener stood trembling.

"What is it, Pram?"

"A snake. A very big one." He pointed to the back garden, his face contorted with fear.

Jean commanded Roxie, "Stay." She stepped out and closed the door. Together, she and the gardener stealthily crept around the back.

The largest cobra she had ever seen lay coiled in the corner of the yard.

Keeping her eyes fixed on it, she told the gardener to get Kissen, their fearless handyman. Her own legs threatened to give out under her as she eyed the monster. She heard Roxie barking, and the noise woke the snake. It raised its head and opened its mouth wide.

"Oh God, let Kissen come quickly."

No sooner had she breathed the prayer than Kissen came, carrying a long bamboo cane. The snake, settled now, had obviously already eaten. With one swift blow, Kissen brought the bamboo cane down into the centre of the coiled body. The snake was no more.

"She had a nest somewhere here," Kissen said. "Most likely in the garage." And without further ado he and Pram carefully removed items and, sure enough, dealt with a nest of baby cobras.

The excitement of the event died down, and a few days later Jean stood in the bungalow that had been her home for over four years, surrounded by boxes and trunks. The moving truck in the driveway heralded the start of her journey back to Reynolds Memorial Hospital.

"This is what you call organized chaos," she announced to Roxie, who whined softly. "You're coming with me, Roxie. Yes you are," she said as she ruffled the dog's coat.

Kissen and Amrut helped the movers load the truck. When the bungalow was finally bereft of her belongings, Jean climbed into the Jeep with a rather bewildered Roxie, and Kissen drove them to Basim.

Jean stood in the living room of the bungalow on the grounds of the Reynolds Memorial Hospital. She had been back in Basim for a week. However, she still yearned for the children she'd left in Chikhli. Roxie, sensing her mood, stood watching her with head cocked as if trying to understand.

"I'm homesick for the children, Roxie. Tomorrow morning, they'll be singing Christmas carols. How I'll miss them." She let out a sigh. Sitting on the settee, she opened her Bible. The dog lay down, letting out her own sigh.

Unexpectedly, Jean's heart leapt as she read the daily scripture. *"And ye shall rejoice in all that ye put your hand unto, ye and your households, wherein the Lord thy God hath blessed thee"* (Deuteronomy 12:7). Peace swept over her and joy flooded her soul. Her devotions finished, she rose with renewed vigour. Startled by her energy, the dog looked up.

"Roxie, I can do all things through Christ, who strengthens me." The dog wagged her tail as if in agreement. "Yes, I can," she said, giving her pet a hug.

"Hello, Jean. I'm going over to the hospital." Doctor Speicher stood in the doorway.

"Right with you." The women walked across the compound together.

"Ranchandra is doing well," the doctor remarked.

"Thank God for that. He took quite a nasty fall," Jean observed. "It's a pity he didn't get to us earlier. Poor little fellow." Memories of her early work flooded her mind. Much progress had been made since those days, and as they entered the hospital she experienced another surge of joy, realizing she'd been a part of it. A physiotherapist was now on staff to treat the young boy.

The missionaries went about the day's business; Doctor Speicher to overview the patients' status and write orders, and Jean, as hospital administrator, to check that all was well on the wards before heading to her office to deal with bookkeeping and schedules.

Sitting at her desk, she wondered how the latest news would affect their work. The Indian government had ruled that missionaries were no longer allowed to own property. This news did not deter the missionaries. They knew God was the ultimate owner. He had allowed the faithful back in North America to raise funds through the years and propagate the work beyond their dreams. Many souls had been saved, and many student nurses had completed studies and become competent senior nurses in charge of the wards. Office staff, maintenance crew, pharmacy assistants and health workers had all trained under the missionaries and many eventually rose to management positions while the missionaries championed them in their roles.

She looked up as someone knocked on her door. "Come in," she called.

Ely, her appointed Assistant Business Manager, entered. "Good morning, Sister. I have completed tallying the money from the Outpatient Department." He held a cash box under his arm and a ledger in his hand. He placed the items on her desk.

With ease, Jean reviewed the columns, checked the totals and smiled.

"Well done, Ely. You'll be in charge before we know it."

Ely beamed. "Thank you, Sister. Thank you." A smile still lit his face as he left.

Jean picked up some papers and concentrated on their content. They were the staffing schedules for the various departments of the hospital. One for the x-ray technicians caught her attention. She noted their hours were not up to par with their pay, and made a mental note to rectify this. Next, she read her memos and checked her planner for meetings. Committee meeting Thursday, district meeting Friday morning, auditors' meeting the following week for the Indian Church, and then several more district meetings.

Completing her office work, she had some lunch, then made her way back to the hospital. Her thoughts turned to the influx of patients diagnosed with tetanus. The moans of a patient disturbed the relative quiet of the afternoon.

"Hello, Sister." The staff nurse in charge greeted Jean.

"How many now?" Jean asked.

"We have seven confirmed cases of tetanus. The doctor in bed five has been touched by the nurses and the fact that they prayed for him."

Jean walked quietly from bed to bed, offering words of comfort and prayer. She stood at bed five. The Hindu doctor looked at her. "Two of your nurses prayed for me last night," he said.

"Yes, so I heard. That's good. Would you like me to pray for you, too?"

The doctor's wife sat at her husband's bedside, looking at Jean with suspicion.

"Whose name will you pray in?" she asked.

"In the name of Jesus Christ." Jean spoke softly. "There is power in His name. Do you see how much better your husband is today? This is a miracle—a testimony to the one true God."

The woman turned to her husband. He spoke. "She is right. I am better, am I not? Come, let her pray for you and me."

And Jean did.

Rounds completed, and one hundred and seventeen patients visited, she went to the bungalow for a brief rest.

"We're here." A few days had passed, and Jean had been to Bombay to have her eyes checked. At the same time, Doctor Speicher had asked her to meet a retiring missionary friend of hers coming from Africa and bring her back to the mission.

"Ann. Lovely to see you. Come in." Hugs and greetings exchanged, the doctor's friend settled in for a three-week stay before travelling home to the states.

Jean's days were filled with juggling her various duties. Missionaries from the Alliance Church, and sometimes other denominations, were guests at the mission. A Japanese evangelist came and spoke with conviction to the nursing and Bible college students. The arranging of sleeping accommodations and meal preparations, with the help of her able Indian staff, were all part of the work.

In April and May of 1972, Jean was still at the hospital, but the unbearably hot weather plagued her once again and she had to leave for the plains. The hospital functioned with a skeleton staff. Jean sat in the railway station waiting for the train to take her to the hill country of Koegall. Her clothes were soaked with perspiration. *It's no good changing,* she thought. *I will wait until evening.* She glanced at her watch. Another five hours. She got up and decided to reserve booking for the return journey at the end of the month. She felt the perspiration trickling down her back and legs while she waited. She downed another bottle of orangeade and then some water. Reservations made, she returned to the waiting room and tried to concentrate on the progress of the work God had ordained for them all.

With a thankful heart, she finally settled on the train and reached her destination. She enjoyed fellowship with Mrs. Sinclair, the widow of an Australian missionary, who ran the guest house. In a letter to her family, she wrote:

June 19, 1972

…Tuesday we went to the Shola Forest; it was simply beautiful. We saw nothing—only birds, and they sang for us. The grey-headed flycatcher, the nuthatch, woodpecker, and other birds I did not recognize.

An American lady drove us by Jeep as far as a home owned by an English lady who lives alone out here. The house is a palace looking out over the mountains and, when clear, she can see down into the valley. This lady was close to the Duke of Windsor's brother. I can't remember his name…She had three husbands and has lived in high circles. There is one son, but he does not communicate with her often. She is alone with her servants and her dogs…it made me sad.

…the air is cold now cold for us. It is wonderful to snuggle in bed to keep warm and get up in the morning before my tray comes, and I take exercise…

The rest over, Jean returned to Basim. She stood with Doctor Speicher, looking out on the dry courtyard. "Even if my seed order had arrived, it wouldn't have done much good. Well, at least the beans from last year are making an effort."

Doctor Speicher spoke. "You know something, Jean, I'm feeling quite homesick."

"Me too," Jean admitted. "But we know everything will work out when we're in God's will. I'll make us a tea," she added, putting the kettle on and taking cups from the cupboard.

Doctor Speicher walked over to the window and looked out at the sparse growth in the vegetable garden. "We have to remember, Jesus said we will reap in due time if we faint not," she said. "So we soldier on. Right, Jean?"

"Yes. Just think of the graduation ceremony yesterday. Twelve graduates, followed by the graduation dinner. We have much to rejoice about and Esther did such a good job with the students, then Carolyn taking care of the catering."

Through August, September and October, the usual downpour of rain had not occurred. The missionaries prayed on. Jean tried to stay focused on the Lord, but found herself worrying at times. Lack of rain affected everything they did. Funds were low, too. Sitting at her desk, brow furrowed, she reviewed income and expenditures, her concentration broken by a knock. Esther poked her head around the door.

"Can I come in?"

"Oh Esther, come on in. I'm racking my brains to find a way out of the hole. We've been in debt for nearly two years now." Jean sighed. "I'm sure everyone's tired of me griping about taking care of supplies. But we are losing on our medicines and we should be doing more charity work than our books show. The outpatient clerk has not made out charity receipts for our charity work. I've had to explain the importance of doing that." Jean pushed her chair back, stood and stretched.

"The times are tough," Esther said. "But God sees all things. I almost hate to tell you this—I just saw the young fellow from maintenance staggering along the corridor."

"I'll have to let him go," Jean said. "I've spoken to him many times. He goes into town late at night and drinks with his buddies. I so hoped he would come to accept Jesus."

Esther spoke softly. "In His time, Jean. In His time. Meanwhile, it's a good system you've developed, paying new people daily wages rather than weekly or monthly."

"Yes, it saves a lot of hassle."

"How are the department heads doing?"

"The x-ray and laboratory heads are getting the hang of it. Our headman in maintenance and his assistant are challenges. I'm praying God will give us a more mature man, one who's steady and organized. The laundry department needs help, too. An ideal arrangement would be a Christian couple dedicated to God and the work of the hospital."

Esther looked at Jean. "Do you want to take a break?"

"A good idea. Let's go over to the bungalow for a tea."

As the women crossed the courtyard, raindrops splattered down. They started to run as the heavens opened, unleashing a torrent. Laughing and almost breathless, they reached the bungalow. Stripping off wet clothes, they grabbed towels and were soon sitting at the kitchen table sipping hot tea and thanking God for the rain.

"I have council meetings to prepare for in a couple of weeks," Jean volunteered. "It's a four-day event, and I've already worked out the menus. What a blessing it is to receive all those food parcels from my sisters, especially the canned meats. You'd be surprised at the dishes we can rustle up with canned meats, curried tuna, curried beef and so on. On top of that, my church family in London sends me cards and letters constantly. I am truly blessed. I better get back to the office for a while. Thanks for the visit, Esther."

"You're welcome."

With a big umbrella and wearing a long raincoat, Jean hurried back to the office. She decided she would work for another hour or so and then write home. She typed a long letter and as usual thanked her sisters for their care and love. Responding to her sister Audrey's question, she wrote:

November 6, 1972

...Audrey asked about my eyes. If God does not heal them before, I am booked to have surgery on my left eye on December 12...at Yadgiri. There is a missionary eye specialist and his wife there, and I will stay in their home. They are wonderful people from the USA Methodist Church. He knows all the new methods...

Geraldine comes back November 22, so will go with me. It is a long story of God's leading thus far, and he has given me several beautiful promises from the Bible, so I always must leave it up to Him to undertake in a way which will glorify Him. If there is no change before our stationing, it will mean that someone will have to be missionary treasurer for at least a while. It would be a strain, so it is wonderful to leave it in His care. It used to be such a big thing, but now it is so simple in comparison to that time. I appreciate your prayers.

Must run now and get Geraldine's bedding roll ready to send with Doctor Speicher when she goes to Bombay. I will go in the car with her tomorrow to shop for council supplies. Then the bedding will be here for Geraldine when she comes in. I think the Andersons will go about the time she comes in, but just in case it will be there. Doctor Speicher is like a little girl getting ready to go away, since she has not been away for so long. She'll have eye and dental checkups.

Love, Jean

P.S. Will doubtless not get a letter off again for a couple of weeks.

By Christmas Day, 1972, Jean's surgery was a thing of the past. She and Geraldine sat on the verandah of Doctor Picard's home after a sumptuous Christmas dinner. Mrs. Picard appeared with three cups of tea on a tray. She spoke to Jean with a soft southern drawl.

"Here honey, you continue to relax. No getting up now."

Jean took the tea. "Thank you from the bottom of my heart. It's been such a blessing to be with you."

"I second that," Geraldine said with feeling.

"The Good Lord has blessed us all," Mrs. Picard said as she placed the tray on a small wooden table before sitting down.

Three days later, Jean and Geraldine returned to Basim. Then, in early January, Geraldine went to Chikhli to be assistant manager at the school. And Jean resumed her duties at the hospital.

On a hot afternoon, she made her rounds on the wards. The rains of the previous year had not been sufficient to ward off a drought. This was the third year of struggle for the whole community. Farmers were unable to plant crops and the government employed many to remove rocks and create roads. This at least afforded a small wage for them.

"Good afternoon, Sister," the staff-nurse greeted her.

"Hello, Nurse. How many do we have now?"

"Eight little boys, Sister. They are all in Ward C."

Jean approached a little fellow in traction. "And how did you break your leg?" Jean asked.

"I climbed the mango tree," he announced.

"Obviously mangoes are a problem as well as a blessing," Jean observed. "It's odd how they do so well in the hot dry season."

The staff-nurse agreed with a nod of her head. "Hopefully these boys have learned their lesson."

The need for hospital care was a constant, and the staff as always did their best to operate on a limited usage of water. But there was always the possibility they'd have to close down for a while if the rains did not come. Jean prayed there wouldn't be any more little boys coming in with fractured limbs.

Rounds completed, Jean walked along the corridor towards her office. Her thoughts flew to Roxie, her beloved dog, who certainly could not live for much longer. There were no vets to consult.

"A penny for your thoughts, Jean."

"Hi, Doctor Speicher. I'm debating what to do about Roxie."

"Well, she is fifteen years old," Doctor Speicher said. "And coughing up blood is not a good sign."

"I know. And I know what I have to do. I'll give her a large dose of sedatives and let her go to her rest. How I'll miss her." She put her face in her hands. Doctor Speicher went to her and quietly placed a hand on her shoulder. Jean Looked up. "Once she's gone, I'll get Kissen to help me bury her in the front. Then, later, we'll plant a tree in her memory."

Doctor Speicher nodded, then gave Jean a quick hug before moving on.

At the end of 1975, Jean went on furlough. She returned to a demanding schedule and more changes, eventually writing a letter to her church family and friends in the spring of 1977 while on vacation.

April 20, 1977

Dear Friends,

It is time for my yearly hot season, in between, Christmas greetings to you while on vacation in the Himalayan Mountains.

A few days ago, as I rode on a local bus about twenty miles around the hills, there before me was the most clear and glorious view of the snow-covered mountains. The Himalayas, like many experiences in life, are rugged at close range, but beautiful from a distance.

With me are many, as yet unacknowledged birthday cards, Christmas cards, and interesting letters. Thank you for remembering me this way, as well as in your prayers. How rich was my furlough, having met many of you and having shared with you the challenge of "building the temple"—His church around the world. The message in 1 Chronicles, chapters 28 and 29, still burns in my heart as He speaks to me. "Be strong and of good courage, and do it." So we can go ahead no matter where we are, because he is with us and meets our every need. Praise His name forever.

Since my return to India last June, the days have been full indeed. I was asked to set up an office for legal and property matters in Buldana. So now I live in Buldana and call it home, while I camp in Washim (formerly Basim) at least ten days a month to help out with hospital administration and midwifery teaching in the nursing school. With all the routine and non-routine, there have been some unusual events.

I arrived back too late to share in the excitement of seeing the film *To Wipe the Tear,* and for the homecoming of many of the graduates from different places who came to say farewell to Doctor Speicher along with the hospital staff. However, I was present when the town of Washim honoured her with a beyond all expectation farewell, for her forty years of service.

Geraldine Chappell and I waved her goodbye at Bombay Airport. It still seems like a dream that she has retired.

Reverend & Mrs. W.J. Anderson—Bo and Mary Ann to us—who retired some years ago, returned for three months and surely they were a blessing as they ministered to us in many ways.

Last month, Doctor & Mrs. Coulter visited. What a rich experience for us in India. They brought with them refreshment, blessings and the challenge of world missions, of which we are a part. Because I live in the district centre, where the assembly was held, I had the privilege to entertain them in my home. It was hot, so you can imagine the amount of food and liquids that was needed for fourteen people for four days. Hilda Moen came from Chikhli and brought ice cubes and cold water—all boiled, of course. Joyce Jakobitz made goodies ahead of time for the breaks. Geraldine and others helped. It proved to be a time of blessing and fellowship to tuck away in our memories.

March 27, Geraldine and I decided not to say goodbye, as she went through the gate at Bombay Airport. She has retired, too. Life has been and will continue to be an adventure for her.

For several weeks before she left, letters and gifts of appreciation were showered upon her, and some from people who were very poor.

Yes, there are hurdles beyond us and heights to climb that seem humanly impossible, but my scripture for this term is Jeremiah 33:3 and God keeps bringing me back to it. We have only praise for Him for what He is doing in the one-year-old baby church in Nagpur. And praise for what He is doing in Aurangabad City, not only in the organized church, but also in the new Aurangabad area where the Peases are now working. Praise for what He is doing in Bombay and other places where the sons and daughters of our village people are holding responsible positions. It is all the fruit of your labour with us down through the years.

As yet the church is small, but we must continue to build until it is beautiful and strong to please and glorify our Master who gave all.

May God continue to bless you.

Sincerely,

Jean Darling

"Thank you for the rain, Lord," Jean murmured as she stood in the office of the Reynolds Memorial Hospital, gazing out of the window. She had finished reviewing the employee provident forms, and waited for Ely, who was now the office manager, to arrive. He entered the office as the phone rang.

"Good morning, Sister," he said as he picked it up. "For you." Ely held the phone out to her.

"Hello." Jean listened with concern to an obviously distressed lady from the Missionary Alliance Headquarters in Akola. One of their missionaries on her way home from vacation had collapsed and died.

"Our problem is getting someone to attend the funeral. Her husband is way up north, and as you know, burial has to take place within twenty-four hours. Can you go?"

"Absolutely. Leave it with me." Taking details regarding the whereabouts of the funeral, Jean told Ely she had to leave.

Doctor Ainscough, one of the missionary doctors at the hospital, stood beside Jean in the little chapel in Akola. The funeral service began. Jean noted the kindness and respect of the Indians who had taken charge of the situation. They had packed the body in ice and then made a simple casket.

The service over, the two missionaries returned to Washim. Jean met with Ely to review some office details, and then headed out for Buldana. Driving along in her car, she reflected on the diversity of her work on the mission field. She smiled. It's books and ledgers, forms and funds, hostess and trustee. Overseeing council meetings and preparing meals for visitors. Sometimes conducting women's Bible studies at the camp meetings, and being a versatile cook and gardener. Her duties took her back and forth to Chikhli as well as other mission stations. She recalled the early days and marveled at the progress made. *I must tell them in my next letter home,* she thought. And so she did.

April, 1978

…At the hospital, God has come with showers of blessings, and The Holy Spirit came quietly and unexpectedly to do a deep work in all of us. A young Indian evangelist came to the Bible school in Washim to minister to the students. They were generous and gracious enough to invite hospital staff, too. Some, who we had been praying for, came to the Master. Victory was theirs. The last morning in Chapel, we did not want to leave His sacred presence.

Nearly all places of leadership at the hospital are filled with Indian staff. They are Doctor K. Meshramkar, Medical Superintendent, Mr. E Bansod, Business Manager, Miss Nalini Yangad, Nursing Superintendent, Mrs. L. Dongerdive, Director of Nursing Education, and Miss Sindhu Gawli, who is in charge of the midwifery department and also teaches the students. We have three fairly new doctors, whom God has surely sent us, as well as all those who do many unseen tasks necessary to the running of the hospital. When Esther Howard leaves next month on Furlough, there will only be Carolyn Myatt and myself as missionaries here.

We pray that God will help every employee to be a dedicated channel that God can work through…

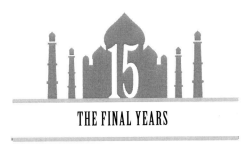

THE FINAL YEARS

O N July 11 of that same year, 1978, a Swissair plane landed on the tarmac at Bombay Airport. Audrey Darling, a teacher of Fine Arts and Music at the Canadian Nazarene College in Winnipeg, and her friend Donna Lee eagerly awaited with fellow passengers to alight. Soon they were going through customs.

"Audrey. Over here." With excitement, Jean waved to her sister. Greeting and hugs exchanged, they made their way to Jean's car.

A whirlwind of activity followed in the next three weeks, with sightseeing excursions, fellowship and meals with missionaries in the district. On the Sunday, dressed in saris, Audrey and Donna went to church. Audrey, through an interpreter, gave the address. In true tradition at the end of the service, the women received a garland of flowers from girls in the congregation. During this time, Jean struggled yet again with a severe bout of malaria, and on occasions could not accompany Audrey and Donna, but was thankful for the warmth and invites they received from missionary friends and staff.

On one of the days when she was unable to visit the sights, Carolyn Myatt filled in. Audrey chose to stay with Jean, and they spent a relaxing day in the bungalow. As Audrey made a pot of tea, Jean remarked, "I'm sixty years old, Audrey, so it's to be expected I can't keep going as much as I once did."

"Yes, that's true, but all through your years here, God has kept you and restored you countless times. Even yesterday we had a great time. Bless you, Jean. I'm thrilled to be here with you."

"And tomorrow we'll be out and about again," Jean said.

And so it was. The visit came to an end, and the women returned back to Canada, with a stopover in Greece along the way, and Jean returned to her work to face more changes.

Government officials in Chikhli had decided that the boarding school was no longer needed. More village schools had opened in the area and the boarders were to be transferred to them.

Jean offered to go and help with selling the school furniture. She set off in her car and moved into a bungalow down the road from the school. The staff struggled with disappointment at the turn of events.

"Think about all the seeds that have been sown here," Jean reminded them. "See how you are testimonies of God's grace. You have all been respected in the villages, people trust you and look up to you, so be encouraged."

The word of encouragement rallied the staff, and they organized teams to supervise sales. Local institutions and villagers came and purchased items. Over a number of days, the job was completed.

All was not lost. The local church started by the Nazarenes, now self-sufficient and run by nationals, took over the property for the district. It served for camp meetings and conferences, remaining a testimony of God's faithfulness to the people of Chikhli.

Jean carried on with a varied and administrative workload. Reading her devotional one morning, she halted—then read again, *Go home to your friends and tell them what I have done for you.* Jean knew God was speaking to her. A tremendous peace engulfed her. She felt no sadness or remorse at leaving her beloved India. God wanted her to continue her work in Canada. Her sister Grace had written to her a few weeks earlier, saying, "Isn't it time you came home?" And so she prepared to leave India in 1984, after forty years on the mission field.

Upon her return to Canada, Jean travelled throughout the country for a year, sharing, preaching and telling of her work in India. At the end of the year, she settled down in an apartment in the house of her sister Grace and brother-in-law. Although it was not really a settling down, but rather an ongoing busyness in her local church, London First, in Ontario, where she served in several capacities. She spoke in many churches and did some volunteer work at University Hospital. A woman of remarkable resilience, she carried on for ten more years. In 1995, she moved into the same apartment building as her sister Audrey.

"Now it is required that those who have been given a trust must prove faithful."
(1 Corinthians 4:2)

"Jean, over here." It was 1988. A large tent had been erected in the grounds of the Reynolds Memorial Hospital, and an even larger number of missionaries to India had returned for a three-day celebration of the hospital's golden jubilee. The tent buzzed with excitement as acquaintances were renewed. Present hospital staff mingled with the brigade that had started it all. Laughter rang out as friends reminisced about some of their improvisation in coping with challenging situations.

Jean waved to Doctor Orpha Speicher, and pushed her way through the crowd to greet her old friend. Geraldine followed behind. "Remember the crow episode?" Doctor Speicher asked.

Over the three-day event, speeches were made, good food consumed, and Carolyn Myatt—now Chairman of the hospital—in her stirring address, said:

...It is our desire that the entire celebration emphasize that everything that has been accomplished by staff, both past and present, was done in the name of Jesus Christ our Saviour, and

Mary Haskett

that it is for His honour and glory we have gathered here. Let us celebrate in this spirit.

"Yes, Lord," Jean whispered, and the words of a hymn that meant much to her came to mind as she stood with the family that had been hers for years and years.

> May all who come behind us find us faithful.
> May the fire of our devotion light their way.
> May the footprints that we leave, lead them to believe,
> and the lives we live inspire to them to obey.
> May all who come behind us find us faithful.
> *Steve Green*